MEDICAL MATTERS IN
VICTORIAN & EDWARDI
WALLASEY

PICTURE POST CARD.

THE ADDRESS TO BE WRITTEN ON THIS SIDE.

AFFIX
½d. STAMP
INLAND.

1 d. STAMP
FOREIGN

This Space, as well as the Back, may now be used for Communication.

(POST OFFICE REGULATION)

Inland Postage only.

FIFTY FREE GIFTS.

Bring this Picture and compare it with those shewn in my Windows.
If it is like either of them in its design,

You Claim One of the Gifts.

GEO. WILSON,

DISPENSING CHEMIST,
403 Poulton Rd., POULTON

☛ Ask for a sample Queen Headache Powder, 1d.

The Address only to be written here.

IF YOUR HEAD IS ALL OF A WHIRL,

and full of aches and pains, you need a "**Queen Powder.**" It will work wonders. They are good enough for a Queen to use, hence are good enough for you.
Prices per packet, 7½d. and 1/-.

IF YOU FEEL LIKE AN OLD CLOCK—

run down by stress and strain of War work, run down to **Wilson** for his "**Tonic Elixir.**" It will wind you up to concert pitch and make you feel as fit as a fiddle.
Price per bottle, 1/-.

IF YOUR LIVER IS SLUGGISH,

and the world looks dull, and life seems a mistake, you need a dose of "**Wilson's S. and L. Pills.**" They will give relief, and you will realise what a beautiful world it really is.
Prices per box, 7½d. and 1/-.

George Wilson was not only a Dispensing Chemist of 403 Poulton Road Poulton but also a 'Marketing Man' ahead of his time! In order to advertise 'Queen Powder' for headaches and his own brands of 'Tonic Elixir' and 'Wilson's S. and L. Pills' he organised a competition in his shop window. Distributing these competition picture postcards locally, if the picture side of the card compared with either of those in his window it entitled the winner to claim one of 50 free gifts (there is no mention of what the prizes were).

Design & Origination
Ian Boumphrey – Desk Top Publisher

Printed by
Eaton Press Direct Westfield Road Wallasey Wirral CH44 7JB

Published by
I & M Boumphrey *The Nook* Acrefield Road Prenton Wirral L42 8LD
Tel/Fax: 0151 608 7611 – e-mail: ianb@wirralpc.u-net.com
for
Dr Richard A Smye

Front cover: Map taken from a Wallasey Local Board Map of 1892
(*Somerville,* site of the present Medical Centre, is pictured below the 'Y' of Wallasey)

ISBN 1-899241-12-4

Price
£5.95

CONTENTS

ACKNOWLEDGEMENTS

Many thanks to the following for their help and encouragement:
My wife, Julie, my parents and mother-in-law; Ian and Marilyn Boumphrey; The staff at Birkenhead Reference Library and Wallasey Central Reference Library; Jane Harvey, Department of Public Health, Wirral Health Authority; Sally Sheard, Department of Public Health, Liverpool University; John Cooper, Wallasey Medical Society; all those involved with the Sabbatical scheme at Wirral Health Authority, for giving me the opportunity to research and write this book and finally to my Partners and all at Somerville Medical Centre.

INTRODUCTION

My intention was to research the development of medicine and health in Wallasey from the early days up to the present day. However I was unprepared for the amount of material and records that survive from Victorian and Edwardian times. I found reading the old, dusty, handwritten minutes of those years became rather addictive and quite fascinating! Some of the episodes written about in these are short stories in themselves and, with descriptions in the language of the day, bring the immediacy of a smallpox or cholera epidemic to life far more vividly than reading a book or printed report about the same subjects. Rather than write about what I found in strict chronological order I have tried to pick out the various strands that I felt ran through these records. I wanted to bring these to life with quotes from some of the sources. The words of the doctors, local people and committees often describe, far better than my words, what life and health meant to those of Wallasey in Victorian and Edwardian times.

I found many unexpected facts, figures and amusing incidents. The visit by the Medical Officer of Health and Inspector of Nuisances to a menagerie in New Brighton in 1878, where they found camels and giraffes, is my favourite of the amusing incidents. As a General Practitioner in Wallasey in 1999, I find the early records of the Wallasey Dispensary, documenting the doctor's work 160 years ago, detail day to day activities that would be familiar to many GPs and patients today. The system developed in the 1830s included asking for a home visit before 10am, being able to see the doctor of one's choice and for some, free health care.

Some of the statistics were surprising, even shocking, to me. Although aware that we are all healthier now, than in the nineteenth century, I had not realised how enormous the difference was. A few examples stand out. Perhaps the most shocking statistic is the fact that if one was a male labourer or artisan, in Liverpool in the 1840s, then one's average life expectancy was 15 years of age. With infection and ill health rife in some areas of Wallasey in the 1840s, even if the life expectancy of this group was better than in the worst parts of Liverpool, lives were being lost at an early age. The numbers of infants and children dying in Wallasey, especially at the end of the last century, from outbreaks and epidemics of infection is, by to-days standards, frightening. Thankfully in the 1990s, we rarely see many of these childhood illnesses, thanks to vaccination and antibiotics. It is easy not to appreciate how disruptive an outbreak of an infection such as measles used to be, before being controlled by vaccinating children. Not only could measles be fatal, but schools had to be closed for weeks at a time to try and control the outbreaks.

Neither had I appreciated what everyday life was like in the last century. In the present time of running, clean water, and sewers that we take for granted, the world of cesspits, night-soilmen and such seem a different world. Indeed, in many ways, it was a different world but due to the single minded determination of the Victorian sanitary reformers, together with local efforts from the Medical Officer of Health, the Inspector of Nuisances and some far sighted philanthropists, these areas were tackled. Drains, sewers, hygiene and housing were improved. Gradually these improvements began to turn around the high death rate that dominated the century. By the end of King Edward VII reign Wallasey was undoubtedly a healthier place than it was at the beginning of Queen Victoria's reign. By 1910 hospitals such as Victoria Central and Mill Lane were well established. Nearly a century later, now combined, Victoria Central Hospital in Mill Lane, continues to be a local asset to us, and has survived the political changes of recent years that have closed so many such local hospitals. Similarly the seeds of general practice, discernible at the Wallasey Dispensary in 1831, have matured into the General Practices and primary care teams that we have in Wallasey today.

Dr Richard A Smye

POPULATION – SOME STATISTICS

The parish of Wallasey ought to be a very healthy district.

Robert Rawlinson, General Board of Health, 1851

The population of the Parish of Wallasey started the nineteenth century at 663 inhabitants and ended the century with around 52,000 inhabitants. By 1910 the figure had increased further to just over 75,000. The rate of increase towards the end of this era was remarkable; the population in 1910 was double that in 1895! The townships increased at different rates over the course of the century. New Brighton's status as a seaside resort saw its population grow from 765 in 1841 to 5665 in 1881. Poulton-cum-Seacombe saw a rise from 380 inhabitants in 1821 to 3044 by 1851, due to the number of industrial works opening in the area. There was a decline in the industries here from 1860 until 1890 after which the arrival of the flour milling industry again drew workers to the area; the population increased almost four times between 1881 and 1910, from around 7,500 inhabitants to 30,000. Liscard township, which included New Brighton, saw the greatest increase over the century, due in part to its larger area and the two ferries at Egremont and New Brighton. Liscard entered the nineteenth century with about 200 inhabitants and had grown to around 28,000 by the turn of the century. Wallasey township itself, Wallasey Village, lagged behind due to its distance from the ferries and poor local transport. The slower growth here meant the population only reached about 4,000 by 1900.

The number of houses obviously increased as the population increased; there were 1,457 houses in 1851 and 10,317 by 1900. The average number of people per house fell from 5.7 to 5.0 over this period. There was local overcrowding but the situation was nowhere near as acute as in Birkenhead. In 1871, for example, there were 607 persons per 100 acres in Poulton cum-Seacombe, 897 in Liscard but 3280 in Birkenhead. The housing in the area ranged from the grand villas in New Brighton to the courts of Seacombe.

Death rates in general in Wallasey did fall significantly over the last half of the century. The worst rate recorded was that noted at the Rawlinson inquiry of 1851 which suggested an annual death rate of 34 per 1000; the figures are only based on what appears to be a particularly unhealthy six months, so are perhaps not an entirely true representation. In 1864 the death rate was 25.6 per 1000; by 1869 the rate had fallen significantly to around 15 per 1000 and the rate remained remarkably constant for the rest of the century, before falling to about 12 per 1000 by 1910. The death rates were reported to the Wallasey Local Board on a monthly basis initially; this reporting started in 1864. There was even debate about having weekly figures submitted at this stage [which would have cost £5 per annum from the Registrar of Deaths] but this was not adopted. Latterly the annual figures were included in the MOH's annual report. The Local Government Board in Whitehall appears to have kept a wary eye on these figures. In 1874 the Wallasey Board received the following letter, questioning a month when there was an unusually high death rate:

Local Government Board
Whitehall
London
29 August 1874

To: T Jones Esq.
Clerk to the Wallasey Urban Sanitary Authority
Egremont
Birkenhead

Sir,
The attention of the Local government Board has been called to the report contained in the Public Newspapers of the monthly meeting of the Wallasey Local Board, from which the following is an extract:
"the number of deaths during the five weeks ending July 29th 1874 was 30, being at a rate of 24.29 per 1000 of population per annum. The number of deaths in July 1872, was 13, being at the rate of 10.53 per 1000 population per annum."
The Board request to be furnished with a Report from the Medical Officer of Health for the Wallasey Urban sanitary District with respect to this very large increase in the death rate of the District, together with any reports he has made to the Sanitary Authority.
I am, Sir,
Your Obedient Servant

J Hepper
Asst. Secretary

There is a note on the letter to say that Mr Byerley, the Medical Officer of Health, had replied but unfortunately there is not a record of his reply.

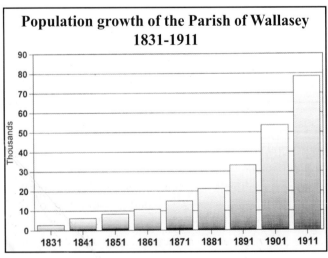

Population growth of the Parish of Wallasey 1831-1911

The graph shows the rapid rise in the population of Wallasey from 2,737 in 1831 to 78,504 in 1911 [census data].

Compared to other local areas, Wallasey had a comparatively low death rate. From 1880 to 1889 the average death rate in Wallasey was 16.40. This compared to a rate of 19.70 for Birkenhead and 23.30 for Liverpool in 1890. By 1910 the difference was still marked –12.9 for Wallasey, 16.3 for Birkenhead and 17.40 for Liverpool.

These average figures, for the whole district, for the year obviously do not show the variation in death rate in various parts of the district. At the 1851 Rawlinson Inquiry Dr Halliday states *In Poulton-cum-Seacombe the mortality is excessive; with all the natural advantages of the locality, it was greater than even in the worst districts of Liverpool; and this opinion was derived from actual experience.* In 1900 the death rate varied from 14.64 in Liscard to 18.95 in Poulton-cum-Seacombe.

The annual rate does not reflect the age of death; the infant mortality, that is children dying under the age of 1 year, can be looked at separately. As Dr Craigmile, the Wallasey Medical Officer says in his 1890 report, *the infant mortality is an important index to the healthiness and sanitary condition of a locality.* While the general death rate declined it was a continuing frustration to the Victorian medical establishment that the infant death rate, nationally, remained constant. Indeed, the infant death rate was actually higher at the end of Victoria's reign than at the beginning, and deaths of infants under the age of 1 years accounted for one-quarter of all the nation's deaths at this time. In Wallasey the infant death rate was 136.4 in 1890, compared to the national level of 151. In 1900 the Wallasey figures were 132.6, compared to 154 nationally. The worst figures for Wallasey were in 1897 when infant mortality reached 168. In that year there were 1265 births and 213 of these babies died before their first birthday. Putting this into perspective today, in 1996 there were 788 births in Wallasey and 6 deaths of children under 1 year of age. If there had been the same death rate in 1996 as in 1897 then there would have been 132 deaths of children under one year alone. 14 children aged five or under died in Wallasey. In 1897 there were 334 children who lost their lives under the age of five.

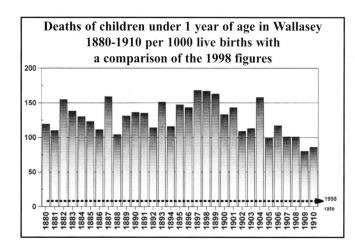

Deaths of children under 1 year of age in Wallasey 1880-1910 per 1000 live births with a comparison of the 1998 figures

During Edwardian times the infant mortality rapidly improved due to a combination of factors, such as better and more hygienic feeding practices and the introduction of health visitors and trained midwives. In 1910 the Wallasey infant mortality rate had fallen dramatically to 86 deaths per 1000 live births.

CELLARS and

OVERCROWDING

I came upstairs into the world; for I was born in a cellar.

William Congreve, Love for love

Dark, overcrowded, stuffy and damp cellars were where the poorest of the population gravitated. Liverpool, in the 1840s, was the worst city in the country for cellar dwellings. Some 38,000 people, one fifth of the city's population, lived in 8,000 cellars. With the poor drainage and cesspits, and privies seeping sewage into the soil, the cellars were, as Anthony Wohl describes them, a form of residential sewer. It was estimated that the death rate in cellar dwellers was 35% greater than the working class in general. Dr Duncan, the Medical Officer in Liverpool, was instrumental in publicising the terrible state of cellar dwellers and in leading efforts to eradicate cellar dwellings. The medical men and local commissioners in Wallasey must have been well aware of the publicity from Liverpool; although cellar dwellers were not as significant in Wallasey, there are references to local problems in Seacombe. Similarly, although there was some local overcrowding of houses, the number of persons per house in Wallasey stayed remarkably constant at around 5.7 from 1851 until 1890, falling to around 5.0 by 1900.

When Robert Rawlinson personally inspected Seacombe in 1851 he mentions *many instances . . . of overcrowding* and that there were unregulated common lodging houses. He does not specifically mention cellar dwellings. There were complaints about an overcrowded house in Seacombe in 1856. In 1858 the Surveyor was asked to report on the *state of the cellars generally in Seacombe.* This followed receipt of an anonymous letter, signed 'A Ratepayer' complaining of the filthy state of premises occupied by Mrs Jones in

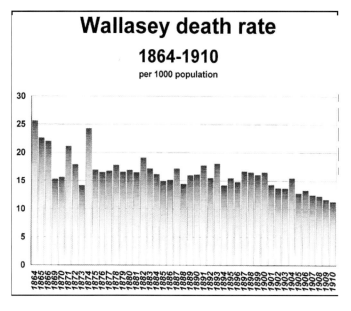

Wallasey death rate

1864-1910

per 1000 population

Victoria Road, Seacombe, where she took in lodgers. Following this inspection the Wallasey Board issued notices *to the owners or occupiers of cellars in Seacombe let separately as dwelling rooms to vacate the same.* Legal proceedings were threatened for noncompliance. Cellars were being occupied in Mersey Street, Seacombe in July, 1865, *in contravention of the Public Health Act 1848 and notices to be served on the owners to cease letting and occupying, within 14 days.* At this time the Surveyor was instructed by the Wallasey Board to give preliminary notices to any owner or occupier permitting overcrowding. He was authorised to *obtain the certificate of two duly qualified medical practitioners in all cases where any such certificate is needed to carry out the provisions of any Act of Parliament for preventing the overcrowding of houses.* The threat of legal action does not appear to have been a great deterrent in this case, as six months later it is recorded that the cellars at Mersey Street were being let again. The 1866 Sanitary Act declared all cellars unfit for human habitation, and in this year the Board prepared a notice to be posted throughout the district *warning persons against permitting houses to be overcrowded.*

However, the practice of letting cellars continued. Three cellars in Abbotsford Street were being used as dwellings in 1871. The Board prepared a poster campaign again, with the following notice to be distributed by placards:

To The Owners of Cottage Property
The Wallasey Local Board hereby give notice that if any house or any part of it be in a filthy or unwholesome condition or that the whitewashing, cleansing or purifying be requisite, or that if any house entertaining more than one family be so overcrowded as to be prejudicial to health, it is their intention to proceed against the occupier of such house with the utmost vigour of the Law.

The last mention of cellars is in 1883; not now used as dwellings but as cellars to shops in Victoria Place, Seacombe. The chairman of the Board urges that a proposed sewer in Victoria Road be commenced urgently *in view of the state of the cellars of the shops in Victoria Place.* If one casts one's mind back, twenty years or so previously, when these cellars were perhaps dwellings, then residential sewer does indeed sound an apt description.

There was some creative moving about of lodgers by some of the owners. There are several complaints of overcrowding that did not appear to be substantiated when the Surveyor or Medical Officer visited. As inspections could not be carried out at night, it seems as though some unfortunate lodgers must have been told to keep away from their lodgings during the day. In 1895 a Wallasey Bye Law was passed enabling inspection of premises at anytime and also gave further powers to regulate the numbers of people occupying each room.

By 1900 the average number of people in each house in Wallasey was about five. There were still some problems with overcrowding. In 1902 the Medical Officer was investigating an outbreak of smallpox in Seacombe when he found 77 people in eight houses. He reports that *they lived in Brighton Place, Seacombe, a blind alley containing eight houses; five on one side and three on the other . . . there is usually no overcrowding in these houses but Brighton Place has for many years been a source of trouble and anxiety to the Sanitary authority, owing to the destructive and filthy habits of its occupants.* Ten of the residents, in these confined quarters, had contracted smallpox.

Overcrowding and cellar dwellings in Wallasey, with their inherent unhealthiness, must have contributed to the spread of infection during this era. Although not as great a problem as in neighbouring Birkenhead and Liverpool, Seacombe in particular reflects the way in which the Victorians viewed, and tackled, overcrowding. The cellar dwellings, in particular, were tangible concentrations of poverty and unhealthiness that the Victorian reformers could fight with legislation and inspection. To the poor, as the population spiralled upwards, overcrowding was inevitable. To the reformers it was an issue to be tackled by improvements in housing, backed by regulations and Acts of Parliament.

By 1910 the situation in Wallasey was noticeably better than 50 years earlier and the developments in housing and reduction in overcrowding had their part to play in the general health improvements at the end of this era.

THE WALLASEY COMMISSIONERS and LOCAL BOARD

Out of the World and into Wallasey

Henry Pooley

In 1845 twenty-one commissioners, residents of the parish, were appointed under a local Act to oversee the *paving, lighting, watching, cleansing and otherwise improving the parish of Wallasey.* There was some medical input to the Commission; one of the Commissioners was Mr John Halliday, a local surgeon and he was present at the first minuted meeting of the Improvement Committee on 9 August 1845. Wilson, in his History of Local Government in Wallasey describes the Commissioners efforts as indifferent and ineffective – *it is on indisputable record that these gentleman took their duties in a cavalier spirit, doing little to improve the district and even that in a grudging and dilatory manner.*

Local residents finally complained to the General Board of

Health in London, in a petition dated 16 June 1851 and signed by Edward Roberts, BA, and 119 others. The signatures on the petition actually included the signatures of several of the Wallasey Commissioners! In response to the petition Robert Rawlinson, the Superintending Inspector of the General Board of Health, visited Poulton-cum Seacombe in July 1851, to compile an *Inquiry into the sewerage, drainage and supply of water, and the sanitary condition of the inhabitants of the township of Poulton-cum-Seacombe.* The Inquiry was held at Parry's Hotel, Seacombe, on 31 July 1851. Dr Halliday was outspoken in his criticism of his fellow Commissioners at the meeting stating that *it is essential that something should be done immediately.* Robert Rawlinson, after personally inspecting parts of Seacombe, published a full report. He covered all the areas of complaint and concluded his report with a strong criticism: *that, as set forth in the evidence, there is a deficiency of local power to grapple with all the evils which exist.* Consequently, in 1853, a Local Board of Health was established, with 15 members. Mr Henry Pooley was elected as one of the members and was appointed Chairman of the Works and Health Committee. His interest in health matters was perhaps sharpened by personal experience. In his memoirs he describes the death of his daughter, Sarah, at

An 1879 advert for Henry Pooley's Iron Foundry and Engineering Company. He was appointed Chairman to the Works & Health Committee.

their house called Gothic Cottage in Seacombe, in the mid 1840s. He attributed her death to defective drainage at the house, which he blamed for the illness and her death. He describes Wallasey at this time – *The whole parish was in a deplorable condition, its rural character spoiled, and nothing done to bring it out of primitive destitution of all things constituting modern civilisation – roads ill-made or unmade, no drainage, no public water supply, no gas works, and its only communication with Liverpool being by ferries altogether worked for private interest without public control, in fact it is justified by a bye word 'out of the world and into Wallasey'.*

With the appointment of a Medical Officer of Health in 1873 the Board could seek, and was given, formal medical advice. There was some criticism of the Board's previous handling of sanitary matters in one of the Local Government Board Inspectors' reports of 1888. The Inspector, a medical officer named Mr Spear, states that *the district has suffered much in its sanitary circumstances from the slovenly operations of the speculative builder and from past neglect of supervision by the Sanitary authority. Of late years, however, there has been a decided change in this respect, and the Sanitary authority, aided now by an energetic Medical Officer and Surveyor, have done much to remedy evils that have arisen.*

Initially there was a combined Health and Works Committee. These separated in the mid 1880s and a separate Health Committee was formed. In 1886 the duties of this Committee included dealing with the night-soil, controlling and managing Mill Lane Hospital and taking the control and direction of the Medical Officer's Department and the Nuisance Department. In 1894 the Urban District Council was created. The Sanitary Department became the Public Health department in 1903.

NINETEENTH CENTURY DOCTORS and THEIR WORK

*If thou couldst, doctor, cast
The water of my land, find her disease,
And purge it to a sound and pristine health,
I would applaud thee to the very echo,
That should applaud again.*

William Shakespeare, Macbeth

At the beginning of the nineteenth century some doctors were both physicians, surgeons and apothecaries. Symptoms themselves were regarded as the disease and there was little understanding of the underlying cause. In the early years of the century the profession began to develop rapidly, with increasing numbers of doctors being trained. The Apothecaries Act of 1815 allowed the Society of

Apothecaries to grant licences for medical practice. In 1838 apothecaries were allowed to charge for medical advice, as well as medicines. By the 1840s many doctors were surgeon-apothecaries; few practised purely as surgeons. These doctors also practised midwifery and were the general practitioners of their day. Until the Medical Act of 1858 created the General Medical Council, as a central body responsible for the training and licensing of doctors, the organisational structure of doctors was confused with at least 19 different licensing bodies.

The Wallasey Dispensary records give a fascinating insight into the employment of doctors by such institutions in the 1830s and 1840s. The doctors were paid 5 shillings (25p) for each case attended; if attending an accident the remuneration depended on the type of accident. The doctors were required to attend the Dispensary daily, except Sunday, at 10am. They were to be remunerated for *prompt attention to cases of malignant cholera*. The rules of their employment, in 1845, state: *In all important cases they shall visit their respective patients at their own home and continue their attendance until they can pronounce such patients out of danger, when they may transfer to the House Surgeon.* It is interesting to note that, even in these early days, the value of a second opinion, in ensuring treatment was necessary, was a written rule: *No important operation shall be performed without a previous consultation from two Honorary Surgeons of the Institution.* The Honorary Surgeon was a man of experience: *A surgeon, having served the full period of seven years, and received an annual vote of thanks, shall become an Honorary Consulting Surgeon of the Institution.*

More people came under the attention of the general practitioner in the last half of the century and unlike today one might see the general practitioner in a number of different ways, dependent on ones' class, income and location. Many general practitioners had part time appointments as Poor Law Medical Officers; others also held posts such as Medical Officer of Health, Public Vaccinators, Port Sanitary Officers and also did work for local hospitals. In Wallasey doctors such as Mr Isaac Byerley and Dr Alexander Craigmile for instance, whose works are discussed elsewhere in the book, held a variety of such posts during their careers. Doctors in towns often had to compete with each other for the various sources of income. Although they may have had private, middle class patients, they often had to depend on other sources of income for their livelihood.

There were a variety of ways in which patients might seek medical consultations. At one end of the spectrum better off families would call the doctor to the house and pay a fee for the visit. In the 1870s and 1880s this might have been one shilling (5p) and by 1910 about three shillings (15p) per visit. The fees may sometimes have been higher. In 1886 Dr Bell submitted an account for £3 five shillings to the Board *for professional attendance to D Gow who met with an accident on 21st May last, while scaling and painting the high level pier at New Brighton.* If admitted to hospital, for instance Mill Lane Infectious Diseases Hospital, the patients' doctor would continue to attend and give medical attention and treatment during the admission. One could pay regular amounts to a Dispensary, such as that in Wallasey or to one of the Friendly Societies, who often employed their own doctors. At the other end of the spectrum, the poor had to rely on medical care provided by charitable organisations or hospitals. Seacombe Cottage Hospital is a fine example of this work, offering free inpatient, outpatient and visits to those deemed 'poor'. These institutions frequently worked at full capacity and had to turn patients away. The choice then was the Workhouse Hospital or, as must have happened all too frequently, the acceptance of being nursed by one's family with fate as the 'treatment'. For many self medication, perhaps relying on

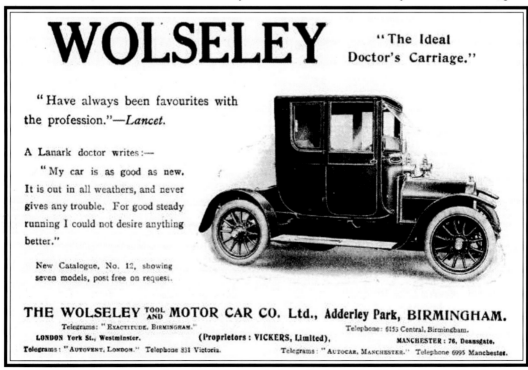

This 1911 advertisement for a Wolseley car is described as *The Ideal Doctor's Carriage.*

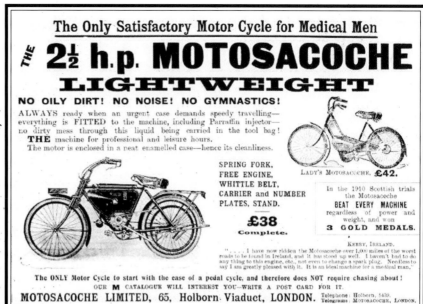

a patent medicine, or advice from family or neighbours, was the first line of help in times of illness.

Doctors usually described themselves as physicians or surgeons, rather than general practitioners. There were few individual doctors' surgeries, such as we would recognise today. It is thus difficult to accurately identify the number of doctors, and their particular work, in Wallasey over the nineteenth century. *Gore's Directory* does list physicians and surgeons and gives some idea of the numbers of doctors in Wallasey over the course of the century; of course some of the doctors listed may have worked in Wallasey and lived elsewhere. In 1829 there is one doctor listed, a surgeon called Mr William Ellis, who lived in Higher Seacombe. John Halliday, a Scottish surgeon, was an active figure between the mid 1830s and mid 1850s. The 1841 census records him living in Higher Seacombe, with his wife and two young daughters. He was 30 years of age at this date. He was one of the Commissioners, appointed under the 1845 local Act, and was highly critical of the Commission at the Rawlinson Inquiry 1851. Other doctors names appear regularly in the various records of the time. Dr Alfred Parr was reporting nuisances to the Board in 1853 and was present at some of the Board meetings in the 1850s. He also consulted at the Wallasey Seaside Institution for Women, in New Brighton, and is noted as an Honorary Consulting Surgeon at the Wallasey Dispensary in 1870. His wife is remembered by Thomas Westcott in his memoirs; in 1859 he recalls Mrs Parr singing *Oh dear what can the matter be* in a room used for penny readings! Dr William Bell, of Rowson Street, New Brighton, was another active medical man. He consulted at Wallasey Cottage Hospital and the Dispensary. He was still active in the early 1900s and is credited with providing the rainfall figures for the Medical Officer's annual report of 1908.

By 1897 there were 32 doctors living in Wallasey. At this time 26 surgeons and 21 physicians were listed, but 12 of the doctors were on both lists i.e. describing themselves as both physicians and surgeons. Doctors' transport was by horse or foot in the Victorian years. With the advent of motorised transport in the Edwardian years cars or even motorbikes were available although doctors would often still visit by foot or bicycle.

Doctors living in Wallasey – Gore's Directory 1897.

Surgeons:

Henry Ambrose Burrows, *Alameda*, Seabank Rd, Liscard
Alexander Craigmile, *Cluny*, Manor Rd, Liscard*
William Crooke, *Glenside*, King St, Egremont

John H. Cropper, 74, King St, Egremont
Wm Cross, *Hope Cottage*, Wallasey Rd, Liscard
John Cunningham, *Lincoln House*, Seabank Rd, Liscard
Alfred H. Godwin, Wallasey Dispensary, Liscard Rd
James Huskie, *Ivor Lodge*, Seabank Rd, New Brighton*
Stewart Kilpatrick, Withens Lane, Liscard*
Stewart McNichol, 110, Brighton St, Seacombe
John Moore, 2, Hillside Rd, Wallasey*
James Muir, *Ellangowan*, Penkett Rd, Liscard
Thomas Napier, *Darlington House*, Darlington St, Egrem.
Andrew Riddell, 114, Victoria Rd, New Brighton*
Alexander Ross, 8, Tregenna Terrace, Liscard Rd, Liscard
Joshua Sanderson, 1, Wallacre Rd, Wallasey*
James Shannon, *Balfron*, Liscard Rd*
Daniel Smith, *Hillingdin*, Seabank Rd, Liscard
John Walsh, *Balrath*, Liscard Road, Liscard*

Physicians:

Alfred Banks, 98 Brighton St*
Wm Banks, *The Bungalow*, Stanley Ave & 28 Rodney St
Wm Bell JP, *Rutland House*, St George's Mount, N B*
Wm Blair Bell, *Linden,* Grove Rd
William Moss Bristow, 2, Falkland Rd, Egremont*
Edward Bennett, *Cratloe Villa*, 95 King St, Egremont*
Alexander Craigmile, *Cluny*, Manor Rd, Liscard*
Wm Cross, *Hope Cottage*, Wallasey Rd, Liscard
John Davidson, *Charemont*, Seabank Rd
John Glencross, 2, Longland View, Rake Lane, Liscard
James Huskie, *Ivor Lodge*, Seabank Rd, New Brighton*
Stewart Kilpatrick, Withens Lane, Liscard*
Thomas Lusk, 131 Victoria Rd, New Brighton
FP Bouverie McDonald, *Ivor Lodge*, Seabank Rd, N B
John Moore, 2, Hillside Rd, Wallasey*
Thomas Napier, *Darlington House*, Darlington St, Egr.
Andrew Riddell, 114, Victoria Rd, New Brighton*
Joshua Sanderson, 1, Wallacre Rd, Wallasey*
James Shannon, *Balfron*, Liscard Rd*
John Walsh, *Balrath*, Liscard Road, Liscard*
* Doctors describing themselves as both Physicians and Surgeons

MEDICAL OFFICER of HEALTH (MOH)

It is the duty of every Urban Sanitary Authority to appoint from time to time a Medical Officer of Health.

The Public Health Act, 1872

In his *Report on the Sanitary Condition of the Labouring Population of Great Britain* [1842] Edwin Chadwick urged the appointment of Medical Officers of Health throughout Britain. The report conclusively established the incontrovertible link between environment and disease. Liverpool was the first city to grasp the challenge with the appointment of Dr William Henry Duncan in 1847. Although the 1848 Public Health Act permitted local authorities to establish local boards of health, few authorities chose to appoint an MOH. In 1872 the Public Health Act made the appointment of an MOH obligatory to all sanitary authorities throughout England and Wales. At that time there were only about fifty MOsH throughout the country. Many local authorities were slow to implement the legislation.

Wallasey was one of the forerunners, and appointed an MOH in 1873, having first discussed the matter in 1865. In 1874 less than half the local authorities nationally had appointed an MOH. The 1875 Public Health Act required medical officers to be registered doctors. The need for further training became appreciated, and in 1886 the GMC formally registered the Diploma in Public Health as a medical degree.

The 1872 'job description' for the MOH describes the wide range of tasks and responsibilities expected of them. These include: being aware of all influences affecting or threatening local public health; being aware of diseases prevalent in the area and on any outbreak of disease 'of a dangerous character' visiting the site of the outbreak without delay; inspecting food; providing an annual report and a quarterly return of sickness and deaths locally; keeping a record of his visits and observations.

Salaries varied. Dr Duncan was appointed part-time in 1847, in Liverpool, on a salary of £300 per annum, with the right to stay in private practice. He soon discovered that the duties were too onerous to be part-time and Liverpool Corporation increased his salary to £750 pa. Others were less fortunate. In 1875 many MOsH earned around £100 pa; in Wallasey the salary was only £50 pa, albeit for a part time appointment, at this date! Out of these salaries many MOsH were expected to pay for their own horses, gigs, grooms and staff.

The MOsH had uncertain tenures. Their tenure and removal was at the pleasure of the local authorities employing them. *The Lancet*, in 1868, questioned the true motives and agenda of some of the members of such local authorities and noted that the government had *entrusted important sanitary powers to local authorities, constituted largely of a class against whom those powers ought frequently to be exercised.*

The MOH worked with a Sanitary Inspector. It was the inspector's duty to make house to house visits, either alone or with the MOH. Much of the routine sanitary work in the MOH revolved around the concept of 'nuisances injurious to health'. These were defined in various Nuisance, Removal and Sanitary acts. The inspector's job was to detect and remove nuisances such as insanitary dwellings, stagnant and foul pools, gutters and watercourses, broken and inadequate privies and ashpits, overcrowded or unhealthy cowsheds, workshops, private dwellings and the like.

The MOH rarely undertook night-time inspections, but their day time visits became a feature of working class life. The inspections persuaded many MOsH that the cause of much disease was poverty. Their annual reports formed the basis for the growing science of preventive medicine.

In Wallasey the post of Medical Officer of Health was first discussed in 1865. Mr Byerley, the local Poor Law Medical Officer was approached by Mr Chadburn, chairman of the Wallasey Board Health Committee regarding the post and on the 28 April 1865 the minutes record that: *Mr Byerley had expressed himself willing to undertake the duties of Medical Officer of Health, without remuneration, for the current year, and stated that at the end of that period both he and the Board would have a better knowledge of the duties required of him and therefore as to what would be a fair remuneration for his services.*

However, the appointment of the Medical Officer is not mentioned again until 1872, so presumably the 1865 appointment was not carried through. In August 1872 the Board received instructions from Whitehall to appoint a Medical Officer of Health; one half of the remuneration to be repaid by Parliament, the other half by the Local Board. In early 1873 the post was advertised, and there were four applications for the position – Mr Byerley, Mr Biggs, Dr W Bell and Dr Pinchin. Mr Byerley was appointed for one year, with a salary of £50. This was on a part time basis. He did apply for an increase in salary on several occasions but no increase was forthcoming!

In January 1881 Mr Byerley gave one month's notice of his resignation and the post was advertised in the Birkenhead News and Birkenhead Advertiser. There were three applicants – Dr Phillips, Dr Davidson and Dr Craigmile. Dr Alexander Craigmile was appointed, again on a part time basis; the salary was still £50 per annum. This was increased to £75 in 1885. Dr Craigmile retired in 1908 and Dr Thomas Barlow was appointed as the first full time Medical Officer of Health in Wallasey. He had previously been Medical Officer of Health for Bootle. He was also a Barrister and was described as a copious writer on sanitary and scientific subjects.

Mr Isaac Byerley

Mr Byerley was one of the leading medical figures in Wallasey for nearly half a century. He came to practise in Seacombe in 1854; this was the same year that his book entitled *The Fauna of Liverpool* was published. This book documents the local fauna and Mr Byerley describes visits to such places as Hilbre Island and Hoylake, to inspect the nets of the fishermen. The expeditions brought to light several specimens which were supposed not to exist in the neighbourhood and Mr Byerley was obviously delighted to report on these. His love of natural history is evident in his introduction to the book:

Strong prejudice has often to be conquered before many can be influenced to touch what they deem 'the unclean thing' and examine the beauty that is hidden under a repulsive exterior.

He lived at Myrtle Cottage in Victoria Road [now Borough Road]. This is described in *The Rise and Progress of Wallasey*:

In the garden was a bowling green and well-stocked pond around which were arranged slabs of sandstone, with the prints of huge extinct Saurian animals, brought from Storeton Quarries.

In her reminiscences of the period Miss Jessie Colley, writing as Miss Dodo in the *Wallasey Chronicle*, remembers fondly visits to Mr Byerley's cottage:

We would run the rest of the way between high hawthorn hedges, only broken by the higher wall which shut in the Earthly Paradise of our doctor. It was not long before we had entered the sacred precincts and been admitted to his consulting room where he had such wonderful stuffed, dried, pickled and bottled creatures; such butterflies, moths and beetles; such jars of clear water containing anacharis and salt isneria; such live creatures as sticklebacks, caddis worms, water fleas and hydras; such a live snake in a sort of box! And we always found him ready to discuss at large on these matters with such genial courtesy that we were almost ready to have a tooth pulled out in order to get there!

She also recalls giving Mr Byerley a great sphym caterpillar as a token of devotion!

He took an interest in local medical matters from the beginning of his time in Seacombe. He is noted as being present at Wallasey Health Committee meetings in the late 1850s and early 1860s. He combined work as a Poor Law Medical Officer with private practice, a common arrangement in those days.

Mr Byerley was appointed as the first Medical Officer of Health in Wallasey in 1873 and he held the post until 1881. He had a long association with the Seacombe Cottage Hospital, from Visiting Surgeon to Honorary Consulting Surgeon on his retirement from active practice. A street was named after him in 1880. Byerley Street, off Borough Road in Seacombe, still exists today. His death, with a fond obituary, was recorded in the Seacombe Cottage Hospital minutes of 1897.

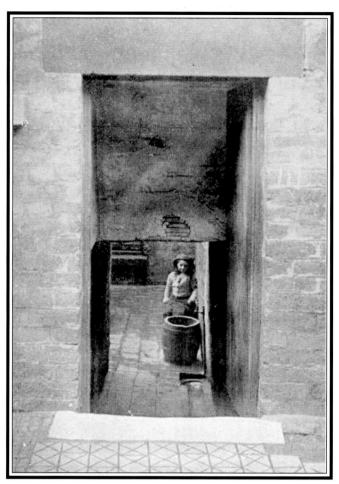

Front view of entrance to common back yard, showing water supply common to two houses in Wallasey. Photograph taken for Wallasey MOH report 1908.

Mr Byerley had submitted handwritten annual reports to the Board; unfortunately these do not appear to have survived apart from his handwritten death rate statistics covering 1866 until 1874. In 1885 Dr Craigmile produced the first printed *Annual Medical Officer's Report.* They make fascinating reading for the medical historian, containing a wealth of statistics and personal observations. The first ten page report, for instance, has detailed figures on the population of the district, births, and deaths, with a specific analysis of infectious diseases. There is also a weather report for the year, supplied by the Bidston Observatory. There is then a detailed discussion of smallpox and typhoid in the area, and also on the state of the drainage and waters supply, with Dr Craigmile's observations and hypotheses regarding these subjects.

As the Annual Reports develop, there are maps showing the sites where infection had been prevalent during the year, and in 1908 photographs illustrating some of the problems with poor housing and sanitation of the time (*see photo on this page*). By 1910 Dr Barlow's Annual Report is over 100 pages long with detail such as a street by street analysis of deaths in the area and comparative statistics with other towns in the area and England and Wales.

THE INSPECTOR of NUISANCES

> *What we call "Progress" is the exchange of one nuisance for another nuisance.*
>
> **Havelock Ellis, 1859-1939**

Until the appointment of the first Wallasey Medical Officer of Health in 1873, there was only intermittent medical input to the Wallasey authorities and much of the responsibility for the population's health, in the wider sense, fell to the Inspector of Nuisances. The post developed from that of Surveyor and eventually developed into that of Sanitary Inspector. These titles were all used at Health Committee meetings, interchangeably, for the post holder during most of the last half of the century reflecting the wide range of his responsibilities.

The post of Surveyor was first discussed by the Improvement Committee of the Wallasey Commissioners in August 1845. The previous post had been combined with that of the Collector and it was decided to separate the two posts. The salary offered was £125 per year and the post proved popular; there were 24 applicants for the job. Mr James West was appointed in September 1845. His main responsibility was to the roads and sewers of the district. He was replaced by Mr Patrick Higgins in October 1848. Inexplicably the salary was reduced to £80 per year at this appointment. The post now had some health responsibilities and soon after his appointment, Mr Higgins was given the remit to take proceedings under the Nuisance Removal and Diseases Protection Act, if needed. Action was prompted, on occasion, by local doctors' concerns. In June 1849 Dr Parr and Dr Donlevy attended the Improvement Committee meeting and raised concerns about the current outbreak of cholera, which they felt was exacerbated by the filthy back streets in Seacombe and Egremont. The Surveyor was instructed and dispatched forthwith to:
remove all filth and noxious matter which may be found, deposited or accumulated in any of the Public Highways or private streets with all justifiable expedition. We know from the Rawlinson Report in 1851 that these instructions were not satisfactorily enforced.

Following the criticisms of the Rawlinson Report Mr Higgins was replaced by Mr Charles Macpherson in 1853. He had previously been assistant to the Borough Engineer in Liverpool. He only stayed in Wallasey for two years. In 1855 he returned to his native Edinburgh as Superintendent of Streets and Buildings.

Mr James T Lea was his successor, appointed in July 1855. He was appointed Sanitary Inspector, under the Nuisances Removal Act of 1855, in August 1856. Mr Lea remained in the post until 1881, although he had a difficult relationship with the Health Committee at times. In 1857 he was asked to be 'more punctual' by the Committee, as he was not always to be found in his offices when expected to be there. By 1863 he needed more staff and was allowed three more road labourers, taking the number of labourers to eleven. He also had two sanitary men and one carter at his disposal; this team was not increased. The labourers were paid 17 shillings (85p) a week at this time. The following year Mr Lea was allowed by the Health Committee, to take on some private practice:
on the understanding that such practice shall not in anyway interfere with the efficient discharge of his duties as Surveyor and Inspector of Nuisances to the Board.
His salary was duly reduced from £250 to £200.

There was a broad range of duties for the Inspector of Nuisances and Sanitary Inspector during the period from 1855–1880. With an increasing population, but only a small team, it must have been increasingly difficult for the Inspector to cover all his responsibilities. There is a distinct impression, from the Health Committee minutes, that the Committee felt by delegating responsibility to the Inspector, usually with instructions that the matter be dealt with immediately, that the Committee had fulfilled its responsibility. Responsibilities included the sewers, roads, contracting for removal of night-soil, preventing overcrowding, disinfecting houses, and from 1873 working with the Medical Officer of Health. The Health Committee's instructions of 1865 illustrate:
that immediately upon being aware of the existence of a nuisance of whatever description [including overcrowded, filthy or unwholesome house] the Surveyor be directed to give preliminary notices to the owner or occupier of the premises upon which the nuisance exists or to the person creating the same, as he may think best to cause it to be removed, remedied or abated to prevent the recurrence.
At this time there was increasing liaison with the local doctors; the above instructions continue:
the Surveyor be authorised to obtain the certificate of two duly qualified medical practitioners in all cases where such a certificate is needed to carry out the provisions of any Act of Parliament for preventing the overcrowding of houses.

In 1871 a sub-inspector was appointed at short notice *the necessity of inspection being urgent, to start Monday next.* Mr Henry Parker was paid 30 shillings per week (£1.50) and provided with a uniform to give an 'official appearance.' [The cost of the uniform not to exceed £5!]. However, in 1874, there were cost pressures on the Inspector's department. The number of labourers under Mr Lea was reduced from 21 to 17 and Mr Lea was again employed on a full time basis. His salary was doubled to £400 on the understanding that he *devoted the whole of his time exclusively to the performance of the duties of his office.* Unfortunately for Mr Parker, the sub-inspector, his services were no longer required, due to the rearrangement of duties.

From this point Mr Lea appears to have had a difficult time.

He was reprimanded by the Board in 1875 for not paying enough attention to his duties in connection with the highways. This reprimand was in response to numerous complaints about the state of the roads. In 1877 'charges of neglect' against him were considered by the Board; these again concerned the state of the roads and also regarding building regulations. The Health Committee stated that *if he wished to regain the confidence of the committee he must bear upon his work with greater energy.*

In March 1881, Mr Arthur Salmon, from Salford, was appointed Surveyor and Inspector of Nuisances with an annual salary of £300. A sub-inspector was appointed again in 1883; Mr Herbert Taylor with an annual salary of £90. During the 1880s there was close co-operation with the Medical Officer of Health, Dr Craigimile. In his annual report of 1888 Dr Craigimile acknowledges the *constant and cordial co-operation of Mr Salmon and the sub-inspector, Mr Taylor, in all sanitary work, both connected with the Hospital and other departments. Mr Taylor's house to house visits and inspections are most useful in detecting defects with drainage, water supply etc.* This was at a time when the Medical Officer was very concerned about the effects poor sanitation might be having on the cause and transmission of infection. An additional sub-inspector was appointed in 1889; the volume of work had increased partly due to the recent Infectious Disease Notification Act and partly due to dealing with increased animal imports from the United States.

Herbert Bascombe succeeded to the post in January 1894. In 1897 the Sanitary Department was formed, with Mr Bascombe as the Chief Sanitary Officer. In 1903 the Sanitary

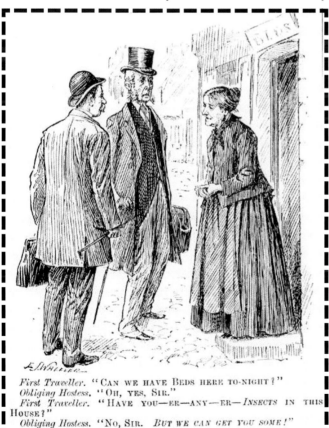

First Traveller. "CAN WE HAVE BEDS HERE TO-NIGHT?"
Obliging Hostess. "OH, YES, SIR."
First Traveller. "HAVE YOU—ER—ANY—ER—INSECTS IN THIS HOUSE?"
Obliging Hostess. "NO, SIR. BUT WE CAN GET YOU SOME!"

This is a 1900 Punch Cartoon.

Department became the Public Health Department. The increasing role in health was highlighted by the appointment of the first Female Sanitary Inspector in this year, Miss Birrell, whose role was that of an early Health Visitor. Her work involved visiting houses, mainly those of the 'poorer classes' and advising on such matters as infant feeding, cleanliness, hygiene and liaison with local schools. She also had responsibility for visiting local workshops where 'female labour is employed'. By 1910 Miss Birrell was visiting 1,771 houses in the year.

NUISANCES

nuisance

n

a person or thing that is annoying, unpleasant, or obnoxious <*found it a ~ getting up so early*>; *specif* an annoyance that constitutes a legally actionable invasion of the rights of another (e.g. to fresh air or quiet)
[ME *nusaunce*, fr AF, fr OF *nuisir* to harm, fr L *nocere*

Nuisance, in Victorian times, covered a wide range of annoyances, some health related and some not. It is a word that is used throughout the period, both by the Wallasey Board in their minutes, and people writing or complaining to the Board.

As described elsewhere the Inspector of Nuisances had an important part to play in Wallasey. There were various Nuisance Removal and Disease Prevention Acts; as the name of these Acts suggest an early link was made between nuisances and disease prevention. The 1848 Act was followed by several revisions over the next 20 years. Nuisances, in legal terms, were such matters as the deposition of 'offensive matter' in or around houses or the overcrowding of houses. A 'short, intelligible complaint of the nuisance' could be made by signature of two householders or by certificate from a medical officer. The Local Authority had the power to enforce the necessary remedy, such as whitewashing or cleaning a house at the owner's expense.

The General Board of Health, in Whitehall, particularly reminded Local Authorities of these measures when there was a threat of cholera and the Wallasey Board received copies and directions about the various Acts. In a circular letter to the Wallasey Board in 1853, signed by the great reformers of the day – Lord Shaftesbury, Edwin Chadwick and Dr Southwood Smith, the Government Board state that *from experience of the working of these Acts that their enforcement operates most materially for the prevention of epidemic disease.*

The complaints of nuisances were almost continually received by the Wallasey authorities throughout the Victorian and Edwardian period. The first documented complaint to the Wallasey Improvement Commissioners was in March

1846 when residents in Wheatland Lane complained about a nuisance being caused by a pit containing drainage water. It would be tedious to document the nuisances recorded, as they run into many hundreds! An extract from the minutes of 6 August 1862 illustrates a typical month's nuisances:

---

6 August, 1862 Nuisance complaints received by Works and Health committee:

Captain Beach, of Wellington Road; of the smell from imperfect drains.

Mr Daniel Shown, of Demesne Street; of manure deposited opposite his back door.

Mr Youds and Mr Peers, of back Church St, Egremont; of the boiling of bones.

Arthur Jackson, of Seacombe; of the Artificial Manure Manufactory

Residents of Liscard; of offal at Mr Leicester's slaughter house

Mr Davidson, Seacombe: of their being no urinal at the *Abbotsford Hotel* and that customers were using his yardgate as a urinal

---

Not all nuisances were health related, although perhaps the complaint about the continued playing of a barrel organ opposite a house in New Brighton, in 1874, would come under psychological harassment these days! Similarly, in 1880, the Inspector had to ensure that steam powered merry-go-rounds on the foreshore at New Brighton, were suitably fenced around, *for the protection of the public.*

Towards the end of the century more nuisances were being actively found than reported. In 1888 the Medical Officer reports. *Some of the nuisances were discovered in consequence of complaints received, but by far the majority were detected by the system of house to house inspections instituted about five years ago.* In 1903 the Lady Sanitary Inspector was still finding *many nuisances* in the course of her house to house visits.

Doubtless in the Wallasey of today, as we approach the twenty first century, we can still find examples of nuisance, but nuisance is unlikely to be as eloquently described as in the hand written minutes of the Victorian Wallasey Board.

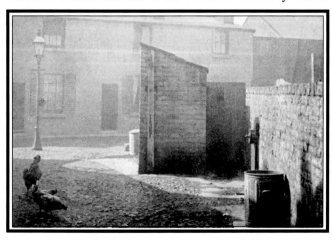

The side of a convenience can be seen in full view of the front of the houses in Oakdale Yard. Note the water supply on the right and chickens on the left – pictured in 1908.

WALLASEY HOSPITALS and DISPENSARY

19th Century Hospitals

Wallasey illustrates the development of hospitals over the century. Voluntary hospitals developed by charitable and philanthropic means. Dispensaries were significant institutions between 1770 and 1850; as with the Wallasey Dispensary they often eventually formed the core of a new hospital. Similarly the small cottage hospitals often evolved into much larger establishments. The Dispensary is an example of a charitable institution giving medical care by the ticket system; the Seacombe Dispensary for Children a charitable institution where not even a ticket was needed and poverty was the only recommendation needed. Wallasey also had examples of fever and smallpox hospitals, which again developed and changed their roles in the twentieth century. The Workhouse Hospital is one institution that was not built in Wallasey. It must still have been a significant institution to the poorest people in Wallasey as many 'paupers' were sent to the Tranmere Workhouse. Even in the early 1900s between 30 and 40 Wallasey residents ended their days there each year.

The Wallasey Dispensary

The Wallasey Dispensary, initially in Littler's Terrace, was a very early forerunner of a local health service. A charity to run the Dispensary was established in 1831. A meeting was held at *Parry's Hotel* in Seacombe on 5 May 1831, chaired by the Rev Alden. It was agreed to establish a Dispensary to offer free medicines and medical advice to the Poor of the Parish of Wallasey. The management was by a Committee comprising of a *President, Treasurer, Medical Practitioner and a Committee of six gentlemen.* The costs were to be covered by charitable donations and also by subscribers. Subscribers of a guinea a year were entitled to receive six printed recommendations for medical attention; these became known as tickets. These subscribers, drawn from the wealthy of the day, were entitled to give these tickets to the 'sick poor'. The rules stated that *the only proper object of the Dispensary being the sick poor, recommended by the Governors of the charity, no person shall, on any account, receive relief who is able to pay for their medicines.* The subscriber had some discretion in this, but generally it was considered those earning more than 15 shillings (75p) per week were not eligible.

The other option was the 6 shilling (30p) subscription, which entitled working men and their families to medical advice and treatment. *Day labourers, tradesmen and others in the*

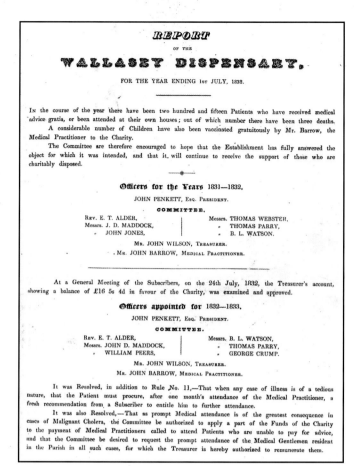

REPORT

OF THE

WALLASEY DISPENSARY,

FOR THE YEAR ENDING 1st JULY, 1832.

In the course of the year there have been two hundred and fifteen Patients who have received medical advice gratis, or been attended at their own houses; out of which number there have been three deaths.

A considerable number of Children have also been vaccinated gratuitously by Mr. Barrow, the Medical Practitioner to the Charity.

The Committee are therefore encouraged to hope that the Establishment has fully answered the object for which it was intended, and that it will continue to receive the support of those who are charitably disposed.

Officers for the Years 1831—1832.

JOHN PENKETT, Esq. President.

COMMITTEE.

Rev. E. T. ALDER,	Messrs. THOMAS WEBSTER,
Messrs. J. D. MADDOCK,	" THOMAS PARRY,
" JOHN JONES,	" B. L. WATSON.

Mr. JOHN WILSON, Treasurer.

Mr. JOHN BARROW, Medical Practitioner.

At a General Meeting of the Subscribers, on the 24th July, 1832, the Treasurer's account, showing a balance of £16 5s 4d in favour of the Charity, was examined and approved.

Officers appointed for 1832—1833.

JOHN PENKETT, Esq. President.

COMMITTEE.

Rev. E. T. ALDER,	Messrs. B. L. WATSON,
Messrs. JOHN D. MADDOCK,	" THOMAS PARRY,
" WILLIAM PEERS,	" GEORGE CRUMP.

Mr. JOHN WILSON, Treasurer.

Mr. JOHN BARROW, Medical Practitioner.

It was Resolved, in addition to Rule No. 11,—That when any case of illness is of a tedious nature, that the Patient must procure, after one month's attendance of the Medical Practitioner, a fresh recommendation from a Subscriber to entitle him to further attendance.

It was also Resolved,—That as prompt Medical attendance is of the greatest consequence in cases of Malignant Cholera, the Committee be authorized to apply a part of the Funds of the Charity to the payment of Medical Practitioners called to attend Patients who are unable to pay for advice, and that the Committee be desired to request the prompt attendance of the Medical Gentlemen resident in the Parish in all such cases, for which the Treasurer is hereby authorized to remunerate them.

This Wallasey Dispensary Report of 1832 also lists the Officers for 1831–32 and 1832–33.

same situation be allowed to subscribe six shillings annually in consideration of which such subscribers and their families will receive medicines and medical attendance without further charge. Midwifery was the only exclusion from this. In 1831 annual subscriptions were £59. seventeen shillings six pence with a total income of £72. There were 41 subscribers of a guinea, and 4 subscribers of six shillings. In the First Annual Report, of 1832, the chairman, Mr John Penkett. reported that *215 patients had received medical advice or been attended in their homes and a considerable number of children had been vaccinated gratuitously.* Patients were required to attend the Dispensary between nine and ten in the morning and to supply their own phials and gallipots for medicines. Patients could ask for a home visit, if not well enough to attend the Dispensary.

In the early days the Dispensary had to deal with the epidemics of the time. In 1833 the Dispensary minutes record that *the committee therefore trust with the blessing of the Almighty, that the prompt assistance afforded to such cases of cholera has proved the means of checking the progress of that fatal disease amongst the working classes and poor of the Parish.* 1840 was a busy year *there were a greater number of patients owing to the prevalence of smallpox and other epidemics.* Medicines were supplied by the Liverpool Apothecaries Co, except in emergency when the doctor could use his discretion to obtain the necessary medicine.

The first 'Medical Practitioner to the Dispensary' was Mr John Barrow. In 1833 two other doctors were also doing work for the Dispensary, a Mr Stone and Mr Willan. The following year Mr John Barrow, Mr John Halliday, Mr William Augustus Barker and Mr William Nesbit were the medical men. They were paid five shillings (25p) per case. The Committee felt it was a good idea for patients to choose which doctor they consulted. *The patient shall, when they receive a ticket, choose the Medical Practitioner whom they wish to attend them, and the ticket must be addressed to the Medical Gentleman chosen; it being understood that each case shall be attended by the person to whom the ticket is addressed.* Dr Freckleton joined the Dispensary as a Consulting Physician in 1834, giving his services gratuitously. In 1837 the Medical Practitioners stated *that it was desirable to make provision for supplying leaches for the poor. In cases where they consider their application necessary it was unanimously resolved to make the best arrangement they could with a decent woman to apply leeches under their direction. The Medical Practitioners are requested to settle with the leach woman and send in their account of her charges.* A leach cost 6d (2.5p) at the time. By 1845 Dr Thomas Hodson was employed as a House Surgeon, with an annual salary of £70. The rules at the time stated that the House Surgeon *shall renounce all private practice and devote himself to the service of the Institution.*

Medical expenses were the largest outgoing for the Dispensary. In 1835 the minutes record that *the sum paid to the medical practitioners considerably exceed the amount of annual subscriptions.* Efforts continued to attract subscribers and by 1839 there were 42 guinea subscribers, including Mr Atherton and Mr Rowson, whose names are synonymous with the early development of New Brighton. There were 39 of the six shillings (30p) subscribers that year. Funds were *sadly lacking* in 1843, so much so that the doctors fees were not paid in full, but owed to them. In this year the six shillings (30p) subscriptions were stopped, and only 4 tickets were allowed for each guinea subscriber. The number of subscribers, and therefore the number of patients, dropped significantly with these changes. The six ticket system was reintroduced the following year, but not the six shillings (30p) subscription. With an increase in donations from church collections, the finances improved. In 1844 the subscription income was £70. two shillings; the income from church collections £101. The number of patients increased again and during 1846 there were 737 patients treated by the Dispensary; 431 of these patients were seen on home visits and 306 patients were seen at the Dispensary.

In 1859 a District Nursing Service was instituted by Mrs Rathbone, of New Brighton.

In 1865 the Dispensary House Surgeon, Mr Churchill, was interested in the post of Medical Officer to the Wallasey Board. The Honorary Medical Officer of the Dispensary informed the Board that Mr Churchill's duties at the Dispensary *were sufficient to occupy the whole of his time.* Drs Nisbet and Parr were Honorary Consulting Surgeons in 1870, with Mr Byerley, Bell and Hammond listed as surgeons and S. Hyde Macpherson Esq. the resident Medical Officer. Ties were developed with the Seacombe Cottage Hospital; as late as 1890 it is noted that the Dispensary Surgeon was providing a daily outpatient service at the Seacombe Cottage Hospital, albeit seeing a fewer number of patients than in previous years. In earlier times medicines had been dispensed from Seacombe Cottage Hospital, by the Dispensary, but by this time patients had to go to the Dispensary to pick up their medicines *a trying ordeal in bad weather.*

There were overtures between the two establishments in 1884 with proposals to unite under one roof. It was not until the early 1890s that the Wallasey Dispensary appointed a committee to look into combining resources with the Seacombe Cottage Hospital to provide a Central Hospital for Wallasey. The discussions came to fruition on 6 July 1899 when the foundation stone was laid for Victoria Central Hospital. The Dispensary continued as a separate institution, under the one roof. It is noted that the Dispensary took up its quarters in the hospital as soon as it was opened. The Dispensary Surgeon was to act for both charities.

Seacombe Cottage Hospital

The origin of this hospital was the Seacombe Dispensary for Children that opened on 1 January 1867 in Fell Street, Seacombe. This was run by a Mr Hammond until November 1869; during his tenure 2,394 patients were attended. In his report of 1869 Mr Hammond declares his belief in free treatment for the poor. *The Dispensary has been quite free, no tickets of admission required, the poverty of the applicant being the only recommendation necessary.* He also describes how important he felt the atmosphere to be, to make the children feel comfortable. *The walls are papered with the coloured pictures issued as supplements to the Illustrated London News and the waiting room is provided with a low table and children's chairs and furnished with some common toys, dolls and picture books. My little patients thus amuse themselves tolerably during the time they have to wait.* Mr Caine of *River View* Seacombe continued the work and he generously erected new premises in Demesne Street which opened as a hospital in October 1871. Adult patients were now admitted; seven beds were initially available. In the first year at Demesne Street 333 outpatients were seen by the Medical Officers; they held clinics three mornings a week. The hospital was funded by charitable donations. In 1872 money was raised from concerts at the New Brighton Assembly Rooms and it is recorded that *old linen and calico are at all times valuable donations. Books, tracts, magazines and castoff clothing, as well as picture books and toys for the children will be most gratefully received at the hospital.*

In 1871, there were 381 outpatients seen as well as 85 inpatients. The various ailments of the inpatients are described thus:
44 medical cases, one of which was brought in dead and 44 surgical cases including one compound and three simple fractures, one strangulated hernia, three burns and scalds, one wound of artery, four incised wound, five contusions and sprains and 21 surgical diseases.

Two new wards were opened in 1885, *many distressing cases having been refused for want of room.* The following year was the busiest to date, with 181 patients admitted.

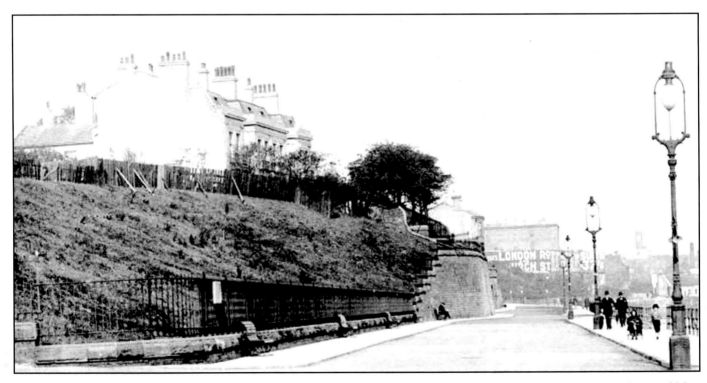

River View, the building on the left in an elevated position overlooking the River Mersey at Seacombe was the home of Mr Caine who paid for the building of the Seacombe Cottage Hospital in Demesne Street in 1871. Out of view behind *River View* was North Meade Hospital (*see page 19*) which is now the site of Wallasey Town Hall.

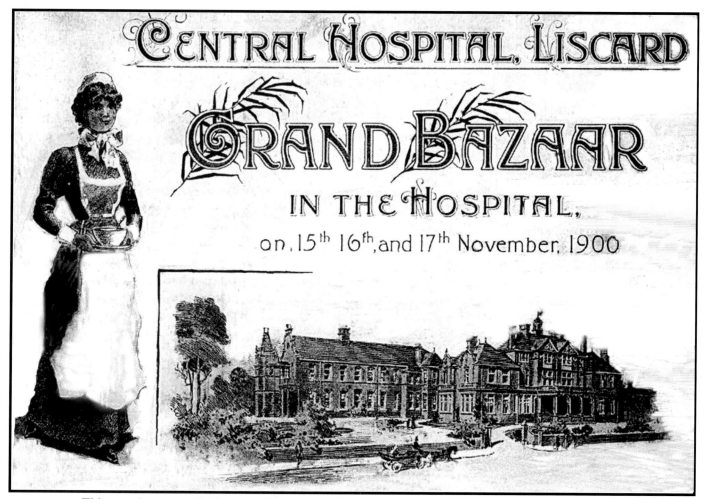

This was the cover of a Souvenir Programme for the Grand Bazaar held in the Central Hospital from 15-17 November 1900 to raise funds for the new hospital.

Following an appeal Mr James Smith funded the services of a District Nurse who was employed in 1886 *to attend to urgent cases of sickness in the homes of the poor who cannot find accommodation in the hospital.* Miss Crilly, the nurse, paid 1389 visits to 65 patients in her first six months.

Communication technology arrived in 1890 and it was proposed *to supply the medical staff with telephonic communication so as to lessen the interval in the arrival of aid in cases of pressing emergency.* The new technology was soon put to use when Dr McDonald provided a horse ambulance wagon which would *when summoned by telephone, bring accidents from any part of the district.*

During the 1890s the pressure on space at the hospital grew, as the local population rapidly increased. There was no space for expansion on the Demesne Street site. The hospital still mainly dealt with the poorer classes. *The poor are always with us and ill-clad, ill-fed and ill housed, they are badly prepared for visitations of disease and accident.* By 1896 the 12 beds were constantly occupied; the daily average was 14 1/2 beds occupied with an average length of stay of 25 1/2 days. The annual cost of each bed was £49. five pence and £3. nine shillings for each inpatient.

In 1897, the Diamond Jubilee of Queen Victoria's reign, the Trustees of the hospital were instructed to realise the assets of the hospital; the £2000 proceeds were contributed to the building fund for the new Central Hospital. When the assets of the Seacombe Cottage Hospital and the Wallasey Dispensary were combined, Victoria Central Hospital was born. After the opening of Victoria Central Hospital on 1 January 1901, Seacombe Cottage Hospital was closed shortly afterwards.

The Seacombe Cottage Hospital premises were sold to the Urban District Council for £1000 in 1901, for use as a Library and Reading Room.

Victoria Central Hospital

Victoria Central Hospital was opened on 1 January 1901. The first patients were admitted at the end of the month. There were 44 beds in this first year; 435 patients were admitted, each staying just over 26 days on average. 646 patients were treated as outpatients

Funding for the hospital was by donation and charitable works. In November 1900 a Bazaar was held by the Ladies of the Parish and the sum of £5400 raised (*see this page for Souvenir Brochure of the Bazaar*). New Brighton Tower Company donated a new Horse Ambulance. X-ray apparatus was purchased in 1903, thanks to a gift.

Eight nurses were employed during the first year; these included four trainee nurses who finished their training in 1904.

By 1910 the new hospital was in full stride and the need for the building of a second pavilion was being discussed.

Wallasey Cottage Hospital

Wallasey Cottage Hospital was founded in 1866 by Mr CC Chambers and was situated in Byron Cottage, Back Lane [now St George's Road]. His charitable aims are recorded in the First Annual Report, written in 1867:

It must be a matter of surprise to those who visit the poor in their homes that people so circumstanced, without good food, pure air, and other hygienic necessities should recover from any serious ailment or accident. Their cottages are for the most part overcrowded, noisy with children, ill ventilated, with windows that barely open, and undrained. These are conditions which depress the vital powers of the strong; how much more pernicious may they be to the weakened bodies of the sick and injured. A Cottage Hospital obviates these evils; it is a place of quiet and rest, clean and well ventilated. It provides good wholesome food and such luxuries as the case of sickness may require; but above all it provides the inestimable benefit of good nursing.

Unfortunately Mr Chambers died soon after the opening of the hospital, so was not able to nurture his project; funds then had to be raised by charitable work or voluntary donation. In 1867 annual subscriptions of £114 were received. In 1903, some 37 years later, it was reported with some disappointment that annual subscriptions had only increased by £19 to £133.

There were two wards initially. Each had two beds, one for men and the other for women. Patients had to pay between two shillings six pence (12.5p) 6d and five shillings (25p) depending on their circumstances. With such limited accommodation, admissions were frequently refused and in 1873 a further 2 beds were made available by alterations to the building; these cost £533 and the hospital was closed for six months while the work was carried out. By 1884 the six beds were always occupied and it was decided to build a new hospital at a cost of £2000. This was opened in July 1886 at a new site in Claremount Road (*see picture below*). A washouse and mortuary were added in 1890. Drs William Bell and Hubbard are listed as the doctors involved at this time.

The hospital remained busy. In 1895 there were 147 inpatients and 605 outpatients. The average number of inpatients was just over ten, with an average stay of 25 1/2 days

The Wallasey Cottage Hospital had a good start to the 20th century with electric lighting and heating being installed. In 1910 an operating theatre, outpatient waiting room, staff bedroom and electric lift were installed. To round off the year the Mayor of Wallasey attended a Christmas Party on 29 December 1910, and kindly contributed a turkey for the Patients' Tea.

Leasowe Smallpox Hospital

In 1899 the Local Government Board made it a condition of a loan for an extension at Mill Lane, that no further smallpox cases would be admitted there. Consequently, several acres of land were purchased adjoining Leasowe Road, at a site deemed suitable due to a sparse surrounding population. In 1902 it was resolved to erect a brick building

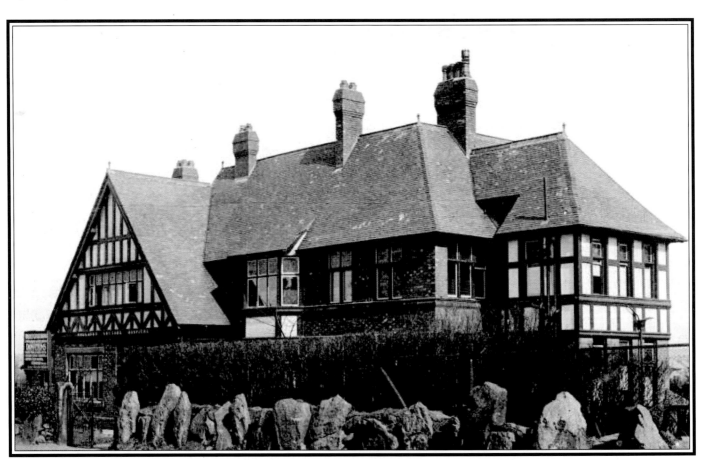

Wallasey Cottage Hospital, Claremount Road,0 opened 1886.

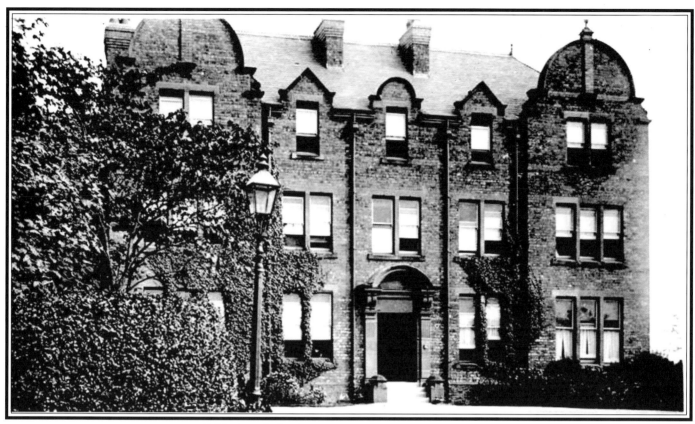

Mill Lane Infectious Diseases Hospital opened 1887.

to house 8 beds. However, an outbreak of smallpox in this year precipitated the swift erection of both a corrugated-iron building, to house eight patients, and also the Berthon tent from Mill Lane to house a further four patients. The corrugated iron building was *lined with wood inside, with the necessary accommodation for nurses and servants, and also a laundry etc.* There were nine beds available in 1906 but, with no small pox outbreak, they were not needed. There was a single admission in 1908; this was a fireman from a ship that had returned from South America.

North Meade Hospital

North Meade House was situated in Brighton Street, where the Town Hall now stands. It was used as an additional infectious diseases hospital in Edwardian times. During the great typhoid outbreak of 1901, when Mill Lane was overrun with 136 admissions, *North Meade* was used to accommodate some of the typhoid victims. It was deemed suitably isolated because it stood in its own grounds. The following year two patients with smallpox were admitted, but it was decided that *North Meade* was not a suitable place to utilise as smallpox hospital. The patients were transferred to Birkenhead Smallpox Hospital while the Leasowe Road site was being prepared. At this time there was also a Reception House at *North Meade*, which was used to accommodate the occupants of houses that had had cases of smallpox. This was a temporary measure while their houses were being disinfected. In 1903, it appeared as though *North Meade* was going to be used for public offices; the possible loss of beds here was one of the reasons used by the Medical Officer of Health to forward a proposal for the building of a new pavilion at Mill Lane. However, *North*

Meade was still being used as a hospital in 1906 when convalescent scarlatina patients were in occupation for several months.

Mill Lane
Infectious Diseases Hospital

The origins of Mill Lane Infectious Diseases Hospital date back to September 1877. The Local Government Board suggested that the Wallasey Board should make *a small permanent hospital into which early cases of infectious disease could be received, if they were not capable of being looked after at home.* As described in the saga of the galvanised hospital *(see page 21)*, the Wallasey Board thought that a temporary hospital would suffice, which delayed the discussion and planning of a permanent hospital.

Mill Lane was proposed as a suitable site in December, 1882. The initial proposal was to combine the hospital with a store yard and stables. The land was owned by the adjacent Grammar School who initially wanted £2400 for the land which the Wallasey Board felt was too expensive. Mr James Smith, of Dalmorton House, Upper Brighton Street, generously offered to buy 10 acres of land, for £2500, and present the land to the parish as a park. At the same time the Wallasey Board bought 3 acres at a price of £1500, for the hospital site. It was a further four years until the hospital admitted the first patient, on 28 October 1887. Dr Craigmile, the Medical Officer of Health reported that there were *many delays and difficulties about preliminary arrangements.* The final building costs of the hospital were £3530. There was perhaps still some antipathy from some of the ratepayers on opening day. Dr Craigmile felt the need to point out that the cost of the hospital would only add 10d (4p) per year to the average house rate. He reminded house owners that with the opening of the hospital, that if any of their servants were to catch scarlatina or diphtheria, then rather than them being nursed in the midst of the family they could now be sent to a *cheerful and comfortable ward, with plenty of ventilation and skilled nursing.* He also reminded the local ratepayers that no-one was immune to infectious diseases:

I look upon the expense incurred [in building the hospital] as an Insurance Premium against the spread of infectious disease, and as we never know how far any given case may spread infection among the community or who may be attacked, it is only right that all should bear the expense.

In his annual report for 1887 Dr Craigmile describes how Mill Lane Infectious Diseases Hospital looked on opening day:
The Hospital consists of three blocks of buildings:
[1] The Hospital proper in the pavilion style, containing four wards, two with three beds each, and two with one bed each. The Small Wards are specially suited for private [paying] patients, for whom a scale of charges has been drawn up. The ground has been laid out so that three other pavilions can at any time be erected.
[2] The administrative block – with kitchen and cooking arrangements, rooms for the caretaker and his wife, sleeping accommodation for nurses when off duty, cupboards for stores, linen presses etc. A Surgery is also provided with a Doctor's room.
[3] Another block containing wash house and laundry, and disinfecting chamber [fitted with a Washington Lyon's Steam Disinfector], a mortuary and a shed for the ambulance carriage.

Local Medical Practitioners were circulated with the conditions and regulations under which patients would be received by the hospital. It was agreed to accept pauper patients for 20 shillings (£1) per week, which included attendance by the Parish Doctors and also ales, wines and spirits! [There were supplies of 'stimulants' at Mill lane – in 1888 brandy was five shillings (25p) per bottle, bottled stout in half pint bottles one shilling six pence (9p). Port wine was also available]. Poor persons, who were not paupers, were to be transferred to the care of the Dispensary Doctor. Others were to be attended by the medical man who was attending the patient's family.

The initial objective of the hospital was to isolate the first cases of an infectious disease outbreak, and *not to house a large number of fever stricken patients.* It was stated that *there are no expectations that the wards will be constantly occupied.* This was not to be the case! In the first two months of being open eight patients were admitted, and one died. With only eight beds and patients being admitted for some weeks at a time, although only 27 patients were admitted in 1888, the Medical Officer reports that the *resources of the present Pavilion have on more than one occasion been already strained to their upmost.* The hospital also received admissions from outside Wallasey. In 1892 three typhoid patients were admitted from the *City of New York* passenger liner; one of these patients unfortunately died. By 1893 the hospital was *repeatedly unable to receive all the patients desiring admission* and the following year a new 12 bed Pavilion was added. More accommodation was needed in 1896 when a four bedded Berthon tent, a canvas structure, was erected as an overflow measure. 1897 was a terrible year for infection in Wallasey, with 120 deaths attributed to infectious disease. Mill Lane was very overcrowded with both ward kitchens used as sick wards at times. 1903 saw the opening of a further 24 bed Pavilion, described as *one of the best and most completely equipped fever pavilions in the country.* Admissions were now about 400 patients per year. With a further 20 bed pavilion being erected in 1905 the hospital now had 66 beds normally, but could accommodate 80 beds if necessary.

Nurses were initially supplied by the Royal Southern Hospital in Liverpool. It was soon clear that a full time

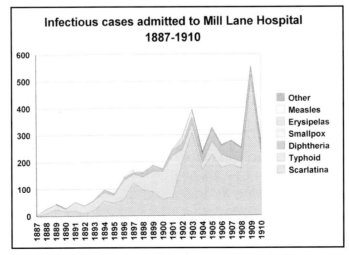

The graph shows the admissions to Mill Lane Infectious Diseases Hospital from 1887, when patients were first accepted. Annual admissions rose from 27 in 1888 to 558 in 1908 with scarlatina, typhoid and diphtheria being the main cases.

nurse was required and a Miss Crilly was employed, at an annual salary of £25. She had previously been the District Nurse at Seacombe Cottage Hospital. The job was not without hazard and Miss Crilly contracted typhoid from a pauper patient in 1890. Shortly afterwards she resigned her post. Typhoid remained a risk to the nursing staff and in the 1901 epidemic, when typhoid was at its worst in Wallasey, and 31 people died from the disease with one of the unfortunate victims being Nurse Hooper. She was a typhoid nurse at Mill Lane; three of her colleagues also contracted typhoid but fortunately had mild symptoms. A monument to Nurse Hooper was erected in Wallasey Cemetery.

Patients continued to be attended by different doctors, according to their class and means. Overall medical control was held by the Medical Officer of Health of the day. Unlike the other hospitals in Wallasey, there do not appear to have been any other doctors specifically attached to Mill Lane Hospital in the early days. Although paupers were treated at Mill Lane, it is apparent that in busy times they were as likely to end up as patients at the Tranmere Workhouse. In 1903, for instance, there were 42 deaths of Wallasey residents recorded at the Tranmere Workhouse.

Lives must certainly have been saved by the efforts of these pioneering nurses, who literally risked their own lives by being in constant contact with all manner of infectious diseases. As there was no specific medical treatment for most of the infectious diseases, the supportive nursing care for these patients was all important. Dr Craigmile says in 1888:
I have no hesitation in saying that several of the poorer patients removed from small rooms where no proper nursing could have been secured would in all probability have succumbed to their illness, had it not been for their removal to Hospital.

THE GALVANISED HOSPITAL of 1877 THAT NEVER WAS!

In March 1877, five tenders were supplied to the Wallasey Local Board for the erection of a temporary Galvanised Iron Hospital. An outbreak of smallpox in the district meant an immediate need for more hospital beds. In April the tender was awarded to Messrs T Morton & Co and a price of £370 agreed. A supplementary tender for an additional room at £37 with an additional £13. ten shillings ten pence for lining the roof with felt was also accepted. The hospital was to be sited on the Board's land at the top of the Breck in Wallasey.

On 22 May, in view of the continued outbreak of smallpox it was decided to proceed with the erection of the building 'at once'. However, on 29 May there was reported to be no

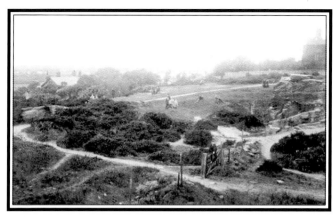

The Wallasey Breck, pictured here, was one of several sites chosen on which to erect the Galvanised Iron Hospital. Although this would have been an ideal site local objections won the day.

suitable place for the erection. The Surveyor was *to urge the contractors to lose not a moment in completing the erection of the Iron Hospital on the Breck.* Such was the urgency that it was agreed that a formal contract be signed with Messrs T Morton & Co, without waiting for the receipt of sanction from the Local Government Board to borrow the necessary money.

By 12 June, however, the Board was running into difficulties due to local objections about the siting of the Iron Hospital. There was pressure from the Local Government Board who had written asking if there was any accommodation in Wallasey yet available for smallpox patients. The Board put forward a proposal to site the Iron Hospital in the shipyard at Seacombe, or on adjoining land. If this was not successful then an approach was to be made to the authorities in Birkenhead with the object of placing the Iron Hospital adjacent to the Birkenhead Fever Hospital. This, it was hoped would be *to the mutual advantage of the Board and the Commissioners.*

On 24 July the Board heard from the Birkenhead Commissioners. *They did not consider the proposal to site the Iron Hospital next to the Birkenhead Fever Hospital should be entertained.* The Local Government Board were still pressing and wrote to express their regret that the Board had not yet found a site.

The locals were still not keen on having the Iron Hospital in their back-yard. On 28 August the Board received a letter from Messrs J Samuelson asking if the Board intended to site the 'fever hospital' in the immediate vicinity of their oil mill at Poulton. The rather curt reply was that no decision to the final site had yet been made. On the same day Messrs Morton & Co requested payment for the Iron Hospital. As it had not yet been sited the Board agreed to pay three-quarters of the amount owing a sum of £315.
By 11 September the Board received another enquiry from the Local Government Board about progress. By then the Board had had enough! They replied that as there had been so many objections to the sites proposed by the Board and that as *smallpox has disappeared from the district* that there was no immediate necessity for the Iron Hospital. They

stated that as the materials had been purchased and fitted together that if an emergency arose the Iron Hospital would `at once be erected.

In October Messrs Morton & Co requested payment of the final balance the Board replied that they soon hoped to be in a position to erect the hospital, and when this was done the balance would be paid.

Messrs Morton & Co seem to have decided to cut their losses and in December informed the Board that they would not be able to erect the hospital for the price named in their original tender.

Things went quiet until the following July 1878. The Board was prompted to look at the Iron Hospital again as Birkenhead Town Council gave instructions that the Birkenhead Fever Hospital would no longer accept patients from outside the Borough of Birkenhead.

They considered several sites including land at the sandhills at the bottom of Grove Road and a site in Green Lane. The Board could not agree a suitable rent and seemed to find a problem with every suggestion. They did not seem keen to finalise the Iron Hospital! This was despite pleas from Dr Byerley. In December 1878 he wrote to the Board reporting that infectious diseases had *prevailed in the Parish during the past four or five months.* He suggested that the Board should take immediate steps to rent some cottages for use as a hospital, or that a wooden erection should be put up as a temporary measure.

Six months later, in May 1879 the Local Government Board was again enquiring about progress. Dr Byerley inspected some land in Green Lane, for sale at £450, which he deemed suitable for erection of the Iron Hospital. Nothing came of this site and the Board contemplated renting some houses in Panama Place but decided the rent of £60 per year was too expensive.

When the Local Government Board again enquired about progress in January 1880 the Wallasey Board enigmatically replied that they *had a site in contemplation.* That was almost the last that was heard about the fate of the iron hospital, as debate about having a permanent fever hospital emerged.

The final mention is eight years later, after the opening of the permanent hospital at Mill Lane. There was a need for extending the accommodation at Mill lane and Dr Craigmile suggested using the material formerly purchased for a temporary iron hospital as an extension. The Surveyor was instructed to obtain quotes, but it is not clear from the Board minutes whether the parts of the old Iron Hospital were used for this purpose, or ended up elsewhere.

FEVER

To all natural evils the Author has kindly prepared an antidote. Pestilential fevers furnish no exception to this remark. I look forward to the time when our courts of law shall punish such cities and villages for permitting any of the sources of malignant fevers to exist within their jurisdiction.

Dr Rush, 18th century American physician

In early Victorian times fever was a word that struck both fear and a certain resignation amongst the population. At the beginning of the 19th century there were few epidemics. Diseases such as diphtheria, influenza and smallpox appeared to be declining. Nobody born in Wallasey during the first two decades of the 19th century, with a mainly agricultural population numbering less than one thousand, could foresee the devastating arrival of infections and epidemics that were to surface on and off for the rest of the century.

The Victorian meaning of fever covered infectious diseases such as cholera, influenza, smallpox, scarlatina, measles, typhoid and typhus. It was not until the end of the century that the cause of most of these infections was discovered. Until then the cause of much disease was thought to be due to spontaneous generation from filth; this was the theory of pythogenesis. This theory suggested transmission of disease was by a noxious invisible gas known as miasma.

It was recognised by the great sanitary reformer Edwin Chadwick, in his Inquiry of 1842, that disease was directly related to poverty, poor housing and insanitary living conditions. Thus began the Victorian thrust to cleanse and sanitise. Worries about the effect of local conditions on health began in the 1840s in Wallasey. The Wallasey Pool was a wide inlet of the River Mersey and when it was dammed up in the 1840s to make the Great Float, a health risk was

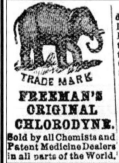

This advert taken from *The Family Doctor and Peoples Medical Adviser of 1891* is for Freeman's Original Chlorodyne. One of its claims is for the treatment and cure of Asiatic cholera, as well as coughs, colds consumption, bronchitis, asthma, sore throat, influenza, neuralgia, diarrhoea, dysentery, colic gout and all fevers. All these cures from only one shilling and one penny (5p) to £1 per bottle!

created and caused great concern to the local residents. In the Seacombe petition to the General Board of Health in 1851 the residents are clearly worried about miasma:

We have to observe that all the drains and sewers from the houses and water closets of the village of Seacombe deposit their filthy contents upon the shore, the stench from which is not only highly offensive to the senses but extremely prejudicial to health . . . a cesspool is formed . . . which engenders malaria, and will in the coming hot season be a fruitful source of fever and disease to a neighbourhood already notorious for its unhealthiness.

There were still similar worries about fevers 13 years later and the Wallasey Surveyor made the following plea to the Wallasey Local Board in 1864:

> 27 May 1864
> *As the hot season is now at hand when fevers and other infectious diseases may be apprehended, special instructions are requested in how to deal with filthy or unwholesome houses, especially in the neighbourhood of Seacombe. These houses are kept by their occupiers in a most filthy state although the owners have, in almost every case, the means of cleanliness.*

The remedy for fevers during the 1850s and 1860s was mainly directed at trying to contain the infection by disinfection of the patient's house by limewashing. In the case of the fevers mentioned above, in May 1864, the Surveyor reported that two houses, where fever was present, had been limewashed. The Wallasey Board had to pay for this and if, as was likely, the occupants were poor the Board was unlikely to recover the costs. With the introduction of the Disinfecting Apparatus in 1875 infected clothing and bedding could be disinfected. The disinfection of houses continued. In December 1879 there is mention of a house in Wheatland Lane being stripped of its paper and disinfected

In the 1870s there was the option to send fever patients to hospital either the Workhouse Hospital or, from 1876, the Birkenhead Fever Hospital. Patients had to pay for their hospital admission. The charges in 1877 at Birkenhead Fever Hospital were three shillings (15p) for each person per day, or part of the day. Patients could apply to the Board for their fees to be paid, on account of poverty and there are poignant lists of such requests. In months such as May and June 1877, 14 requests for payment of hospital fees on account of poverty, were received and accepted by the Board. These fees varied from 18 shillings (90p) to £7. sixteen shillings. Some were not so lucky as the following entry illustrates:

26th June 1877 Letter from I Pratt, dated 5th instant, asking for some consideration on account for the amount charged to him for maintenance of his wife at Birkenhead Fever Hospital and for disinfecting his bedding, amounting to £6. two shillings nine pence. The Board recommended that one half the amount be allowed, and that the remaining half be paid by instalments of five shillings (25p) per week.

There were also beds at the Wallasey Cottage Hospital and Seacombe Cottage Hospital, but these were often full, particularly at times of an epidemic. Mill Lane Infectious Diseases Hospital admitted its first patient in late 1887. Disinfecting facilities were also established here.

Many infections 'visited' Wallasey in the nineteenth century. Smallpox is the only one of these to have been totally eradicated since then. Other infections, such as scarlet fever and typhoid, can now be treated with antibiotics. Others, such as measles, diphtheria and whooping cough are kept at bay by vaccinating children. We are wise to remember how things were before these developments. If resistance to antibiotics grows, or the number of children being vaccinated falls, we may ourselves again experience the old fear of fever. Let us hope not.

This is a Lever's advertisement dated 1892 which includes a nurse's letter recommending the use of 'Sunlight' Soap during a cholera epidemic.

Cholera

The birth of the first cholera epidemic to ravage Wallasey was in Jessore, India in August 1817. This was a new disease, Asiatic cholera. Fifteen years, and many thousands of miles and deaths later, cholera reached Seacombe and from here quickly spread to Liverpool. The first case of Asiatic cholera in Great Britain was in Sunderland, Co Durham on 25 October 1831. Despite the efforts of the Central Board of Health in London to contain the outbreak, cholera defied all known and conventional precautions and so the spread was inevitable and unstoppable. Cholera was declared in Liverpool 12 May 1832. By the time it had run its course across Great Britain over 30,000 people had died.

Cholera returned to Wallasey a further three times. In June 1849 two local doctors, Drs Parr and Donlevy attended the Wallasey Improvement Committee to express their concerns about the epidemic, and urged the Commissioners to improve local sanitary conditions.

27th June 1849: *Dr Donlevy and Dr Parr having attended the committee stated that there had been several cases of Asiatic cholera within the parish, particularly at Seacombe, several of which had terminated fatally and that the habitations of many of the poor at Seacombe were in a very filthy and unwholesome condition and that many of the back streets required to be cleansed. The Law clerk was requested to prepare a notice to be printed and issued by the Head Constable on the occupiers of such cottages requiring them to whitewash, cleanse and purify the same.*

Two years later, at the Rawlinsinon Inquiry, these fears were repeated, little having been done in these intervening years. Mr Richard Parry stated that *if something be not done, and that soon, many people in Seacombe will be suffering from fever and cholera, as before.* There were further outbreaks in 1853 and 1866.

During these further epidemics, the General Board of Health in London issued precautionary advice to the Local Boards. In 1853 the Wallasey Board received such advice which optimistically stated that cholera is *not so suddenly fatal as is supposed* and that if proper medicine is applied that the disease would usually be stopped. Later bulletins received by the Board in the 1870s were more realistic. There was still debate over the treatment of cholera amongst the medical men of the day. Remedies that were tried for cholera included moderate bleeding with leeches, warm baths followed by flannel rubs, a mixture of castor oil and

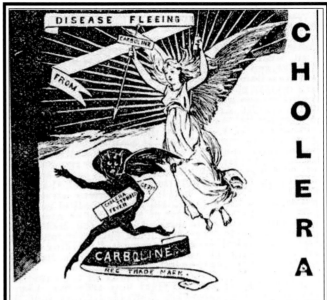

Ellison's Carboline was a disinfectant against Cholera seen in this 1892 advert in *The Family Doctor.*

laudanum and plasters of mustard, peppermint and hot turpentine.

Patent medicine purveyors had a field day with concoctions such as Daffey's elixir, Moxon's Effervescent Magnesium Aperient, Morrison the Hygienist's Genuine Vegetable Universal Mixture, Freeman's Original Chlorodyne (*see advert on page 22*) and Ellison's Carboline (*see this page*).

The cause of cholera, the bacillus cholera vibrio, was not found until Koch's work in 1883. However, it was established in 1854, by Dr John Snow in London, that cholera was spread by infected water supplies and the improvement in the general sanitary situation over the last half of the century lead to the virtual disappearance of cholera by the end of the nineteenth century.

The eyes surrounded by a dark circle are completely sunk in the sockets, the whole countenance is collapsed, the skin is livid . . The surface of the skin is now generally covered with cold sweat, the nails are blue, and the skins of the hands and feet are corrugated as if they had been long steeped in water . . . . The voice is hollow and unnatural. If the case is accompanied by spasms, the suffering of the patient is much aggravated, and is sometimes excruciating .
George Bell, Edinburgh surgeon. Writing of his experiences with cholera in India in the 1820s.

Smallpox

Smallpox was the only major disease to be contained and turned back by medical discovery during this period. Vaccination against smallpox was discovered by Jenner in 1798. However, it took nearly 100 years for smallpox to decline. In 1840 free vaccines were offered to anyone who requested vaccination. In 1853 a compulsory Vaccination Act was passed which made it obligatory for parents to have their children vaccinated within three months of birth.

The uptake of the vaccine was sporadic, even after a further law in 1871 imposed a fine of 25 shillings (£1.25) on those who refused to have their children vaccinated, with imprisonment for non-payment of the fine. The numbers of babies vaccinated actually fell over the last quarter of the 19th century; by the end of the century only one in four babies were vaccinated, compared to more than nine out of ten in 1875.

In Wallasey smallpox is mentioned and discussed frequently at the earlier Wallasey Board Health Committee meetings. There was a national epidemic of smallpox from 1870 until 1873, in which some 44,000 people died. This affected Wallasey particularly in 1871. In February 1871 the Wallasey Board discussed the outbreak of smallpox in the district with the Birkenhead Board of Guardians and concluded *that everything was being done that was requisite in the matter.* They decided it might be advisable to *appoint a person to watch and warn persons against going in and out of, or near to, premises where persons were suffering from the disease.* The Surveyor was authorised to appoint such a person, but by the end of the month he reported that smallpox was on the decline and so this person was not appointed.

Smallpox returned to Wallasey in 1876 and 1877 and this outbreak first prompted the Wallasey Board to contemplate a fever hospital. At the start of the epidemic in 1876 the Board was keen to remove smallpox cases out of the area, rather than provide local facilities. In July 1876 they were informed that a patient with smallpox from Poulton, had been removed to the Workhouse Hospital. They looked into the 'power of removal' and found that, under the Public Health Act of 1875: *any person who is suffering from a dangerous infectious disorder, if not in suitable lodgings, or on board ship, may be removed by order of any justice, on a certificate signed by a medical practitioner.* Further, if the person removed was a non-pauper any costs were to be borne by the patient, or his estate if he died. Smallpox continued to be epidemic in Wallasey during 1877; in May 1877 the Surveyor reported that since September 1876 there had been 53 cases of smallpox and that 12 had died. At this time there was thus a one in four chance of dying from smallpox once it was contracted, so the fear of the disease is understandable. The Surveyor reported that *in all cases disinfection of the premises, where sickness had occurred, had been promptly attended to, and the bedding and clothing that was infected or suspected of infection had been promptly purified, or in some cases destroyed.* He stated that all cases had been referred to the MOH. Smallpox is not mentioned again until January 1884 when the MOH attended the Health Committee in person. He stated that: *a serious case of smallpox had occurred in Waverley Street, Seacombe and that he had done all he could in the absence of hospital accommodation in the district . . . to prevent its spread by having all who lived in the house removed, except for the mother of the sick man.* This particular case has two happy endings, the following month it is reported the man had recovered from smallpox and had been paid £2 compensation for his bed that had been destroyed. It was noted that his bedding had been thoroughly disinfected and had escaped incineration!

In January 1886, the Surveyor reported *that there had been a bad case of smallpox at Seacombe. The patient, Mr Phillips, of 59 Edgmond Street, had died and that he recommended that the bedding used by him, which was estimated to be worth £1. thirteen shillings four pence, should be destroyed.* The Board agreed to pay the relatives this amount, in compensation.

Wallasey was almost free from smallpox during the 1890s but in 1902 the local doctors were forewarned by an epidemic in Liverpool, which had spread to Birkenhead. Some of the younger doctors had not seen smallpox before and some early case were thought to be chickenpox. In that year 39 people caught smallpox.. There were seven cases of smallpox in 1910, including the three year old daughter of one of the disinfecting staff. Dr Barlow, the Medical Officer of Health was concerned about the declining number of children being vaccinated. In 1885, 99% of children in Wallasey were vaccinated against smallpox; by 1910 this had fallen to about 75%. Each child should have been vaccinated in four places. Parents tried to avoid their children having the full vaccination. Dr Barlow states about a local medical practitioner: *as a matter of fact I know that a very*

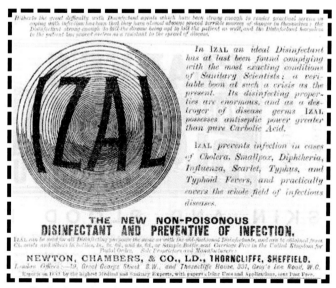

Izal advertises in 1893 that their product prevents infection in cases of cholera, smallpox, diptheria, influenza, scarlet, typhus and typhoid fevers. This was then one of the more reliable disinfectant products.

large number of infants in this district are taken to a neighbouring town [presumably Birkenhead] to be vaccinated, because it is notorious that a certain gentleman in that town will meet the parents in the most handsome manner, and allow them absolute discretion in regard to choosing the extent of the vaccination of their children.

Typhoid

Tyhoid fever is caused by salmonella bacteria and is spread by eating contaminated food or drinking contaminated water. People can become carriers of the disease, and remain infectious for months or years. These sources of the typhoid bacillus were not recognised until this century. It is an unpleasant infection, causing incapacity for two or three weeks, and if untreated proves fatal in up to 25% of cases. There was a significant typhoid problem in Wallasey at the end of the last century; looking at what the local doctors felt might be the cause, and the extent of the problem, is an interesting insight into the Victorian thoughts on the cause of disease.

Dr Craigmile, the MOH from 1881 to 1908, was exasperated by the continuing cases of typhoid during his tenure. He initially supported the accepted theory at the time that typhoid was caused by a noxious gas or miasma. In his 1885 report he stated that *I have had the best reason to believe that in former years cases of typhoid originated from sewer gas entering houses.* The following year he again discussed the origins of typhoid commenting that *sewer gas of itself is not dangerous but suppose it contains the germs of typhoid then what happens when it is freely inhaled in passing a manhole?* In his 1888 report he comments *the typhoid fever poison may make its home, there is every reason to believe, in the soil – the poison once finding its way by leaky drains or otherwise into the soil is likely, under favourable circumstances, to reassert itself.*
It was clear that typhoid could spread from person to person, but this was perhaps not realised by the general public. In describing the spread of typhoid in a family in Oakdale Road in 1887 Dr Craigmile says *all these instances show the folly of supposing that typhoid is not a contagious or infectious disease.*

There was general resistance amongst doctors of the day to accept that polluted water was the source of infection, but Dr Craigmile did consider this cause while investigating a fatal case of typhoid in Wheatland lane in 1889: *there was a strong possibility of the disease having been got from water drunk from a foul ditch in the country. In this case a friend of the man who died stated that he saw bubbles of gas rising from decomposing matter in the bottom of the ditch and would not himself drink any of the water.* In the early 1890s he did not accept that typhoid could be caused by infected drinking water or milk. However, in 1899 his interest in discovering the source of typhoid led him to visit North Wales to inspect the milk supplies, but he did not find any definite evidence of typhoid. He details an investigation of a typhoid outbreak in Rankin Street and Limekiln Lane this year, which was attributed to a blocked

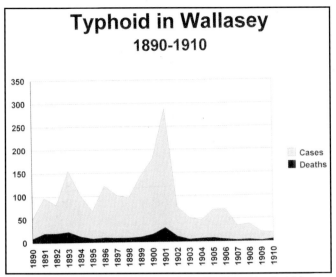

This graph shows cases and deaths from typhoid in Wallasey 1890–1910.

sewer. He concluded that:
the infected excreta from one or two of the early cases had lain in the blocked sewer and there, with the high temperatures, had found a favourable breeding ground.

He inspected the milk supplies again, in 1900, and samples were examined for the typhoid bacillus; it was now clear that this was the offending organism but in this case no infection was found in the milk. It was becoming clear to Dr Craigmile that typhoid could be caused by food: *In the autumn of 1900 some cases of typhoid were reported having in common that all these persons had attended a banquet and all had partaken of oysters. One of these typhoid cases was fatal. I was able to ascertain where the oysters were procured, and learned that they were dredged from beds in Dublin Bay close to which a large portion of the sewage of Dublin Bay is said to be discharged.* It became clear that people were also contracting typhoid from eating cockles and mussels collected from the Wallasey shore. Boards were erected on the shore to warn people of the dangers.

Typhoid was at its peak in Wallasey in 1901 and Dr Craigmile was clearly upset and disappointed in having to report 257 notifications of typhoid in this year, with 31 deaths. He estimated that up to 55% of these cases were caused by infected milk; again he visited farms in Cheshire and North Wales. In 1906 there were 65 notifications and five deaths but after this, as in the country as a whole, typhoid rapidly lessened in incidence in Wallasey. In 1910 there were 14 notifications with five deaths. It was still a dangerous infection but Dr Barlow was able to state that:
I think that it can be truthfully be said that typhoid is a disease that is rapidly disappearing in England.

Typhoid was a barometer of inadequate water supplies and sewerage. Despite it being unclear to those at the time that these were the sources of typhoid, the general drive to improving these amenities led to the reduction in typhoid. Dr Craigmile's efforts to improve Wallasey in these areas were eventually rewarded.

Various Infections

Scarlet fever

Scarlet fever, otherwise known as scarlatina, was a devastating childhood infection in its day. Like so many other infections the cause was unclear during the Victorian era, but it became clear to the authorities that early isolation of infected children could hinder the spread. It was established this century that scarlet fever is caused by a bacteria, spread by close contact between children. *It is a quite usual thing amongst the poorer people when a child is taken ill, for it to be removed to the kitchen or the living room and if the disease happens to be scarlet fever, that of course means everyone in the house is exposed to infection* reports Dr Barlow in 1909. The infection was more deadly in the last century than nowadays. The bacteria itself was perhaps more virulent then and combined with poor nutrition and overcrowding could be deadly. In the 1880 epidemic, which affected the country, it is estimated that 1 in 5 children who caught scarlatina died from the infection.

In Wallasey scarlet fever was a major cause of concern in the early 1860s. There was a discussion about scarlatina deaths in July 1863. The Board decided to monitor the situation by obtaining a weekly list of deaths in the parish from the Registrar of Deaths at a cost of £5 per annum to the Board. There were 58 deaths from scarlet fever between September 1863 and January 1864 and Poulton-cum-Seacombe seems to have borne the brunt of these. With the population being about 11,000, many families must have

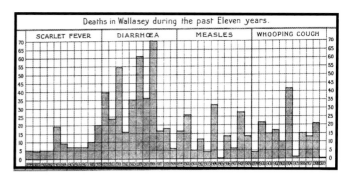

This chart lists the deaths due to scarlet fever, diarrhoea, measles and whooping cough in Wallasey from 1899–1909.

been affected by this epidemic. 1863 appears to have been the worst year for fatalities from scarlet fever. For the rest of that decade there seem to have been on average one or two deaths per month. In 1889 the infection was noted to be *more than usually fatal and prevailed during the greater part of the year.* There were 18 deaths this year. From 1890 the death rate from scarlet fever fell dramatically. In 1890 one in ten children who caught scarlet fever died; by 1910, when there were only three deaths for the year, less than one in 100 children with scarlet fever where dying. Towards the end of the century scarlet fever was still prevalent and virulent enough to cause outbreaks of infection. Substantial numbers of children were admitted to Mill Lane Hospital. In 1900, for instance, there were 119 cases of scarlet fever notified. Half these cases, 60 in number, were admitted to Mill Lane.

Compulsory notification of diseases such as scarlet fever was introduced in Wallasey in December 1889; this would have helped the enforcement of isolation of infected children. Parents were prosecuted for failing to comply. Dr Craigmile outlines the procedure in his 1890 report :
On a case being notified to the MOH, the name, disease and address is handed over to the Sanitary Inspector. The Sub-Inspector visits the house and ascertains various particulars. The Head of the School attended at once receives information and also the School Attendance Officer, so that children from an infected household are prevented from attending school.

Measles

Measles is another infectious illness that used to cause disruption to schools and deaths amongst children. *No infectious complaint spreads with such rapidity among children* observed Dr Craigmile. In epidemic years there were a significant number of deaths from measles. In the epidemic of 1887 there were 29 deaths from measles. Ten years later there were 34 deaths. Some of the local schools were closed for up to six weeks; The Infant School in Union Street dwindled from 90 pupils to 15 pupils at the height of the 1887 epidemic. Dr Craigmile felt there was *gross carelessness on the part of parents and guardians in letting children suffering from measles mix with healthy children.* Schools were often closed due to measles outbreaks, to prevent spread of the illness. In the period from 1897 to 1900 schools were closed for four weeks every summer for this reason. In 1910 there were still 15 deaths from measles.

Statistics re Scarlet Fever since 1881.

Year.	Estimated Population at Middle of Year.	Total Notifications.	Attack Rate per 1,000 of Population.	Percentage of Cases removed to Hospital.	No. of Deaths.	Death Rate per cent. of Cases.	Death Rate per 1,000 of Population.	No. of Cases Admitted to Hospital.	No. of Deaths in Hospital.	Percentage of Deaths in Hospital to Admissions.
1881 ..	21,192 (Census)	..	..	..	..	..	..	..	..	..
1882 ..	22,743‡	..	..	..	29	..	1.27	..	..	..
1883 ..	24,037‡	..	..	..	21	..	0.87	..	..	..
1884 ..	25,228‡	..	..	..	5	..	0.18	..	..	..
1885 ..	28,000	..	..	..	4	..	0.14	..	..	..
1886 ..	29,500	..	..	..	4	..	0.13	..	..	..
1887 ..	30,500	..	..	..	8	..	0.26	..*	..	..
1888 ..	31,500	..	..	..	1	..	0.03	10	..	..
1889 ..	32,500	†	..	..	15	..	0.43	25	3	12.0
1890 ..	34,000	116	3.4	14.6	12	10.3	0.35	17	2	11.8
1891 ..	33,500 (Census) 33,229	89	2.6	20.2	7	7.8	0.21	18	1	5.5
1892 ..	34,500	49	1.1	18.4	3	6.1	0.09	9	1	11.1
1893 ..	35,500	123	3.4	17.0	2	1.6	0.06	21	1	4.8
1894 ..	37,000	246	6.0	22.7	5	1.0	0.13	56	..	..
1895 ..	39,000	130	3.3	36.1	4	3.0	0.10	47	2	4.2
1896 ..	41,500	157	3.7	38.2	4	2.5	0.09	60	3	5.0
1897 ..	44,000	256	5.8	48.0	15	5.8	0.34	123	7	5.7
1898 ..	46,800	220	4.7	44.1	11	5.0	0.23	97	7	7.2
1899 ..	49,000	167	3.4	53.3	5	3.0	0.10	89	3	3.3
1900 ..	52,000	119	2.3	50.4	4	3.3	0.08	60	2	3.3
1901 ..	54,000	147	2.7	45.5	5	3.4	0.09	68	4	5.9
1902 ..	55,000 (Census) 53,579	293	5.3	67.9	5	1.7	0.09	199	4	2.0
1903 ..	56,000	440	7.8	70.2	18	4.1	0.32	309	11	3.5
1904 ..	57,000	270	4.7	62.9	8	3.0	0.14	170	7	4.1
1905 ..	58,500	348	5.9	62.0	6	1.7	0.10	227	3	1.3
1906 ..	62,000	266	4.3	66.9	6	2.2	0.09	178	6	3.3
1907 ..	67,000	255	3.8	73.7	6	2.3	0.08	188	6	3.2
1908 ..	71,000	248	3.5	70.1	10	4.0	0.14	174	9	5.1
1909 ..	73,000	716	9.8	70.8	20	2.7	0.27	507	14	2.7

* First Case in Hospital, October 28th, 1887 (7 to end of year).

† 1889 Notification Act adopted December 2nd, 1889. (30 Scarlet Fever Cases notified to end of year).

‡ These figures are for the end of the year.

Scarlet Fever statistics from 1881 to 1909.

Diphtheria was also called 'throat fever', 'malignant sore throat' or 'inflammation of the throat'. As with scarlet fever the percentage of those contracting diphtheria who died was very high. Diphtheria was fatal to one in every four or five children contracting the infection. Until 1860 diphtheria was listed with scarlet fever by the Registrar General. In 1883 the diphtheria bacterium was discovered and in 1894 an anti-toxin was introduced into general use; Dr Craigmile refers to these discoveries in his 1894 report: *it is only quite recently that it has been possible to recognise true diphtheria by microscopic examination of the secretion, which contains a bacillus or germ characteristic of the disease. There are good grounds for hoping this terrible disorder will be rendered far less fatal in the future by the use of a substance known as antitoxin.* His optimism was well founded and the use of the anti-toxin lead to a significant fall in the death rate from diphtheria following its introduction.

As with the other illnesses there are no accurate figures for diphtheria in Wallasey until 1882. There is mention of deaths from diphtheria in the 1860s, but only at a rate of one every few months. Perhaps some of the deaths attributed to scarlet fever were actually caused by diphtheria at this time, due to the confusion between the two illnesses. In the 1880s there were between three and nine deaths a year, so diphtheria did not have as great an impact as some of the other infections. The numbers of deaths remains similar through the 1890s and early 1900s, but as the population had grown rapidly the actual death rate from diphtheria had fallen. In 1900 Dr Craigmile was able to state *prompt treatment by the injection of diphtheria antitoxin has been most beneficial in saving life from this disease.* This infection must have been terrifying for children and parents alike; in 1906 six patients, including a four year old, needed emergency opening of their wind pipe, a tracheotomy, to relieve the blockage caused by diphtheria, at Mill Lane Hospital. To help promote the use of the anti-toxin, arrangements were made in Wallasey, in 1910, so that anti-toxin could be obtained 'free of charge' by any medical man requiring it.

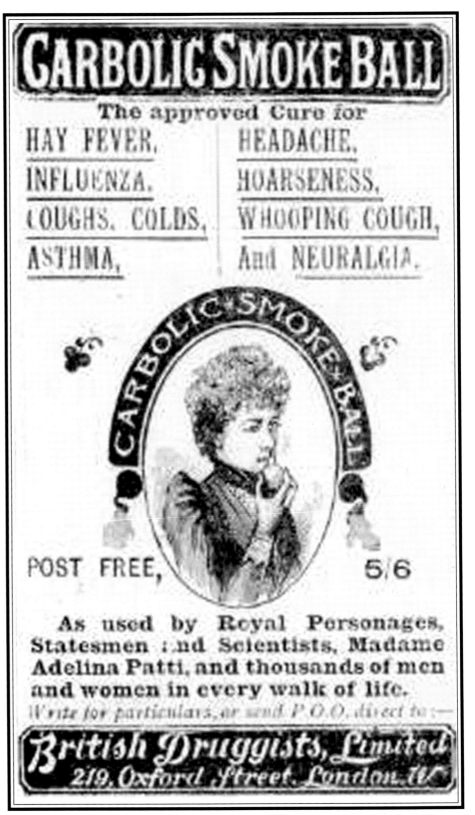

Whooping Cough was one just one of many illnesses cured by the Carbolic Smoke Ball which the lady in this 1897 advert seems to be inhaling from. It seems very expensive for then priced at five shillings six pence (27.5p).

Whooping Cough caused serious epidemics in Wallasey; again not much mention is made of this infection prior to 1882 but this was probably due to it being simply categorised as 'bronchitis'. There is still no effective treatment for whooping cough over 100 years later but thankfully it is now rarely seen due to effective vaccination. In 1885 there were 18 deaths from whooping cough. Dr Craigmile's observed that:

whooping cough pure and simple is not a serious disease but there is always a tendency for bronchitis to set in. Hence we see that among the poor of Seacombe, where the children are not well looked after and where the houses are colder and the means of warmth scantier, the fatality is much greater than among the Liscard population.

Whooping cough continued to cause significant numbers of deaths during epidemic years; 22 deaths in 1900 for example. Many school days must have been missed during the outbreaks. Dr Barlow, the Medical Officer of Health for Wallasey, issued an advice leaflet for the parents of children with whooping cough. This advised keeping children off school for at least six weeks and suggested that *the child suffering from whooping cough should be put by itself, and a fire lighted in the room. If this is impossible, every parent should see that the child does not go out into the street, and that other children are not allowed in the house. Infected rooms should have their windows thrown widely open for two or three days after being occupied by the patient.*

Diarrhoea was another cause of the demise of many

young children. Nationally it was the single largest cause of infant deaths in the 1890s. This was reflected in Wallasey; from 1895 until 1900, there were an average of 77 deaths a year from diarrhoea. Although deaths from diarrhoea declined sharply in King Edward VII's reign it still remained a major cause of infant deaths. In Victorian times the diagnosis of diarrhoea, as a cause of death, did not specify the underlying cause, which was often unknown. Most of the fatal cases of diarrhoea would have been due to viral or bacterial infections, made worse by such factors as the baby's general health, sanitary conditions at home and poor feeding. There were outbreaks of 'infant diarrhoea' which today would be recognised as due to a viral infection; it was observed these outbreaks were worse during spells of hot weather. Also to blame for the large number of deaths was poor feeding of babies. Despite Victorian doctors condemning artificial feeding this remained a potent cause of illness. Babies might be fed with infected cow's milk or even condensed milk. The baby's bottle might be an old ginger beer bottle and the teat could have been made from India rubber. The poorer families could not afford these and continued to use old rags or cloths for the purpose, a recipe for the breeding of infections.

As the causes of diarrhoea became clearer after 1900, so local authorities encouraged promotion of breast feeding and education about hygiene for mothers. Health visitors were employed to do this work. Thus in Wallasey a Female Sanitary Inspector was appointed in 1903 and most of her duties were those of a health visitor. In her 1903 report she describes her work in this area:
Enquiry visits during the autumn were paid to houses where fatal cases of Infantile Diarrhoea had occurred and in almost every instance the method of feeding was found to be incorrect. A great amount of ignorance still prevails on the subject of infant feeding. Special enquiries are always made at the time of the visit as to the method of feeding, and instructions in such cases is given verbally, together

with a printed memorandum on the care of infants and young children. It has been found in many instances that these leaflets have borne good fruit and that the advice given by the Female Inspector has been acted upon with good results.

In 1910 Dr Barlow, the Wallasey MOH, discusses the merits of breast feeding in preventing illness; in his enquiries he found that of the babies dying under the age of one year, twice as many were bottle fed as breast fed.

Tuberculosis [TB], also known as consumption

or phthisis, was the greatest cause of death, from disease, in Victorian times and is estimated to have accounted for about one third of such deaths during this era. Early statistics are unreliable as it was often confused with bronchitis or other illness. It was an infection that particularly affected those who were poorly nourished and living in cramped conditions. It was recognised that in confined quarters the infection was easily caught, particularly if in contact with infected spit. Dr Craigmile first discussed TB in detail in his 1897 report: *Again the terrible fact that 70,000 persons, at a very moderate rate of calculation, die every year of this disease has forced the prevalence of Tubercle not only upon the minds of medical men, but upon all men and women who take an interest in the welfare of their fellows. It is also calculated that one in ten of the Population suffers in one form or another from Tubercle.* He also reminded the local doctors of their duties:
Meanwhile it will not be out of place to mention that it lies largely with Medical Men to help by giving instructions about the disinfection of all expectoration from Consumptive patients. Dr Barlow returns to the subject of TB in his 1909 report. He noted that the death rate from TB in Wallasey was much below that in the rest of the country. He felt that the rate amongst long standing Wallasey residents was even lower due to the influx of people from outside the area Such people, he noted, came to Wallasey as *the good reputation of this district attracts people suffering from phthisis to come and live here, in the hope of improving their condition.* One third of deaths from TB that year occurred in people who had been resident in the district for less than 12 months. Dr Barlow carried out a detailed analysis of TB patients; details such as occupation, alcohol consumption and the patients' 'habits' are documented.

Typhus, also known as Irish fever, gaol fever or putrid

fever was an infection mainly spread by the faeces of the body louse. Mortality was high with about one in three people, who contracted the infection, dying. It was much less prevalent in Wallasey than Liverpool and the last death from typhus recorded in Wallasey was 1878.

Accurate figures are not available, but between 1863 and 1869 there are only seven typhus deaths recorded in the Health Committee records, suggesting that even at this stage typhus was not of major significance locally.

DISINFECTION

It is to cleanliness, ventilation and drainage, and the use of perfectly pure drinking water, that populations ought mainly to look for safety against nuisance and infection. Artificial disinfectants cannot properly supply the place of those essentials.

John Simon, Chief Medical Officer, 1866

To the Victorian establishment cleanliness was paramount in preventing and tackling infection and disease. Disinfection was the usual response to outbreaks of disease and involved whitewashing of houses and disinfection or destruction of clothes or bedding. There were instructions from the Government Medical Department in 1866 describing how to sterilise rooms with chlorine gas, nitrous acid gas or sulphurous acid gas! Quicklime was the most usual disinfectant used for general disinfection either as a powder for sprinkling on offending areas or dissolved in water for disinfecting clothing.

In Wallasey quicklime was frequently used. In 1865, for instance, the Surveyor purchased two bags of chloride of lime and was sent forth to *cause houses in an in a filthy or unhealthy state to be whitewashed, cleansed or purified.* The quicklime was also used to 'disinfect' ashpits and cesspits. When houses were disinfected this often involved the stripping of wallpaper, as well as whitewashing. There was discussion about using carbolic acid for disinfecting the streets in 1871, but this was deemed too expensive. The disinfectant requisition for July 1885 is an example of the items used, and their prices:

Chloride of lime	Ten shillings per cart
Sanitary oil	two shillings nine pence (14p) per gallon
Carbolic acid	
Special No 4	three shillings (15p) per gallon
Ordinary No 5	Two shillings six pence (12.5p) per gallon

Disinfection of clothing and bedding was first carried out at the Disinfecting station at the old Gas Works in 1875; in 1887 a new Washington Lyons Steam Disinfector was installed at Mill Lane Hospital. There were frequent claims for compensation for clothing that had been disinfected. In October 1888 a Mr JH Tyson of 85 Bell Road Seacombe claimed £3 compensation for damage to a fur coat! He was compensated with the sum of £2. five shillings.

In 1885, 41 rooms in 33 houses were disinfected along with 432 articles of clothing and 38 beds. The work seemed to ever increase; by 1892 there were two disinfection vans, one for taking articles to the disinfecting station and one for returning the articles. Rooms were now being disinfected

Right: Condy's Fluid advertisement of 1911 claims an amazing variety of uses – from being used in post-mortems and dissections to an antiseptic mouth wash or an injection in gonorrhoea!

with sulphur fumes. 84 rooms in 69 houses, 1216 articles of clothing and 223 beds and mattresses were dealt with this year. The disinfecting work continued apace in Edwardian times. By now 'formalin' was also being used as a disinfectant in houses where there had been cases of tuberculosis.

In 1910 Dr Barlow, the MOH, was rather sceptical about disinfectants and there was some disquiet amongst the residents when he ended the practice of using disinfecting powder when bins and ashpits had been emptied. He puts his views in no uncertain terms: *It has more than once been prophesied that the stopping of the practice of throwing this disinfectant powder promiscuously about would have very serious effects on the public health. These prophesies as you will have found on reading the preceding pages [of the annual report] have altogether been falsified. The public are so inundated with advertisements of disinfectants, as to what they will do [there is nothing they will not do], that the practice of disinfection is in danger of falling into disrepute. The usefulness of disinfectants is strictly limited, and when they take the place of soap and water and cleanliness, as I fear there is danger of their doing, their use is fraught with grave danger. Disinfectants in the hands of ignorant people are quack remedies. Many of them are themselves useless, while others, which may be good, are rendered useless by their manner of use [see advertisement for Condy's Fluid on previous page].*

Even so, disinfection by the Sanitary Department showed no signs of slowing that year with 386 houses, 7847 articles and 100 books from public, private or school libraries being duly disinfected!

The Disinfecting Apparatus

In February 1874 the MOH, Mr Byerley, asked the Board to consider:
the desirability of the Board having an apparatus for disinfecting by heat, which apparatus might be used promptly in all cases where diseases occurred which had tendency to spread by infection.
In support of this proposal he presented a communication from Dr Trench to the medical profession in Liverpool, urging the provision of such a facility. The Board did not take the matter forward until nearly a year later when the MOH again wrote, drawing attention to
the necessity of providing a disinfecting apparatus for preventing the spread of infectious diseases, by stoving bedding, clothing, carpeting etc.
The Surveyor was instructed to look into adopting a room in the Water Tower, to site the apparatus. He visited the Birkenhead Workhouse, 'an establishment in Liverpool', and also discussed the matter with the Liverpool Inspector of Nuisances. An estimate from Messrs Tessimont & Kassick for £110, for the disinfecting apparatus was accepted but Mr Kassick condemned the idea of using the

Water Tower and an additional £35 was needed to house the apparatus. A site was found on spare land, owned by the Board, at the Gas Works in Poulton Road.

There was an objection in October 1875 from Messrs J Samuelson & Co about the erection near to their works and they wrote to the Local Government Board (*see below*).

Local Government Board   22 Fenwick Street
London   Liverpool
       October 18th, 1875

Sir,
    We regret to be compelled to seek your protection under the following circumstances. The Wallasey Commissioners have, notwithstanding our respectful remonstrances, opened a shed with an apparatus for disinfecting infected clothing in almost immediate contiguity to the gate of our Oil Mill, West Float, Poulton.
    We have a considerable number of men engaged upon work continually passing in and out besides persons coming to and fro on business. That the Board consider the place dangerous is obvious from the fact of their having put the entrance to the shed as near as possible to our gate and as far as possible from their own.
    We can obtain no satisfaction whatever from them, their reply to us being that their Medical Officer of Health has approved the site and that they have no other suitable land in the Parish.
    We have no wish to stand in the way of desirable sanitary arrangements, but we feel sure you will agree with us that it would be better to burn infected clothing than to deal with it in a manner calculated to jeopardise the lives of labourers.
    Your obedient servants,
    James Samuelson & Sons

However, the Medical Officer *did not consider that any evil consequence could arise from its osition and that he knew of no situation better suited for it, than that chosen, insomuch as it is one in which dwelling houses are never likely to be built and where free circulation of air is always maintained.*

In January 1876 the Local Government Board insisted that the Disinfecting Apparatus be housed in an enclosed yard, which was erected at a cost of £50. A van was also purchased for conveying infected clothing to and from the Apparatus.

Messrs Samuelson & Co must have regretted suggesting incineration as an alternative. In May 1878 a memorial from the employees at Messrs Samuelson & Co was received, complaining about the smell from the incineration, and conveying worries about the health risk to themselves.

The Medical Officer investigated and concluded:
that it is probable enough that unpleasant smells might arise from the combustion of materials of which flock-

bedding, blanketing or clothes are composed but that no fear of infectious diseases might be apprehended from such a cause as disinfection would take place during the process of burning.

Despite these reassurances it was decided that it would be preferable for the incineration to take place in *some place remote from dwellings and burn them in the open air.* It is not recorded where this place was found!

Working with the Disinfecting Apparatus must have been an unpleasant job. Clothing and bedding was heaped into an iron steam chamber for about five hours and the smell and heat from this, and the incinerator, can be imagined.

A Mr Davies, employed to attend the Apparatus, asked for a pay rise of two shillings (10p) per week but this was refused. Unfortunately the job appears to have driven him to drink and in February 1877 he was suspended for being repeatedly intoxicated on duty.

The Apparatus was used 31 times in 1885 and was still in use in 1887. In August of that year the Surveyor was asked to report on the practicality of using the Disinfecting Apparatus for the burning of diseased animal carcasses. This was prompted by the need to dispose of two diseased sheep carcasses.

With the opening of the new Washington Lyons Steam Disinfector at Mill Lane Hospital later that year, it is likely that the Disinfecting Apparatus at the Gas Works was superseded.

CESSPITS SEWAGE and SMELLS

In no town in England is there more actual filth and all that may produce disease than in certain portions of the comparitively rural village of Seacombe.

Robert Rawlinson, General Board of Health 1851

Of all the factors in the high death rate from infectious disease in Victorian times, none was more important than faulty or inadequate sewerage. As the population grew these inadequacies threatened to submerge towns in large human dung-heaps of their own making. Wallasey's experience of the increasing problem was typical of many areas of the country, the problem increasing as the population expanded.

There were several phases, progressing intermittently at times, in the gradual improvement of the situation in Wallasey over the course of the century. In the first half of the century cesspools were the most common form of excrement disposal. As the population grew these became choked and saturated land and contaminated nearby wells. The cleaning of cesspits was such an unpleasant task that local authorities hesitated to tackle the problem, as described in the chapter about the night-soilmen. At this time, as quaintly described in the *Rise and Progress of Wallasey*, it was usual to answer the 'call of nature' wherever that call came and to follow the habit *not uncommon in rural communities of regarding every stream or creek as a sewer provided by Providence.* The letter from householders in

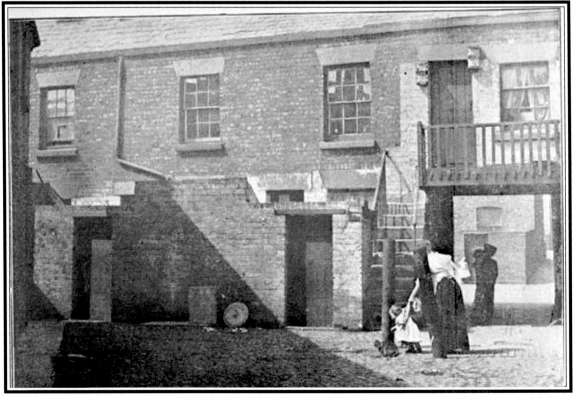

Victoria Court, **mentioned above in Rawlinson's report of 1851, was of a similar design to *Oakdale Court* Demesne Street Seacombe, pictured here in 1908. Although over 50 years later, when much of the squalor had gone, the grim features of this type of development remained.**

Poulton-cum-Seacombe to the General Board of Health in 1851 states that *all the drains and sewers from the houses and water closets of the village of Seacombe deposit their filthy contents on the shore, the stench from which is not only highly offensive but extremely prejudicial to health.* The smell would have been combined with that of middens and privies adjacent to houses. The privy midden was little better than a small, private cesspit but not all houses even had this luxury. In 1865 there are still reports of new cottages being built in Seacombe without privies or water closets.

Robert Rawlinson, when he personally inspected Seacombe in July 1851, provides a fascinating eye witness description of some of the unhealthy sites. One can almost smell his following account of visiting Victoria Court, which was behind houses in Demesne Street, Seacombe (see photo on opposite page of Oakdale Court, Demesne Street).

This court is entered by a narrow covered passage; the court forming a square, without proper means of ventilation. In the centre are privies, and a large cesspool, which receives the refuse from the surrounding inhabitants, and here it remains for months at a time, generating poisonous gases. The whole atmosphere of the court at the time of my visit was very offensive, and, according to the best medical testimony, must have been most prejudicial to health. I was informed that the owners of this property had expended £130 in trying to improve and drain it; but in consideration of the street sewer not being laid at a sufficient depth, this money is wasted. I never inspected a court in a worse sanitary condition. Fever is common amongst the inhabitants, and cholera had prevailed. There is a slaughter house and pig-meat boiling establishment not far distant, which are described as a great nuisance.

There was obviously a temptation for the authorities to deny these unsavoury problems. In 1874 the Surveyor inspected a cesspool and could not detect anything more disagreeable than the sight of the place. The alternative was to use one of the heaps of manure in the road, frequently mentioned

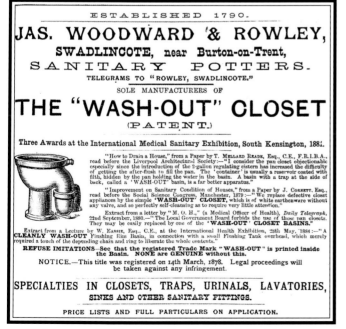

This was an 1890 advert for the 'Wash-Out Closet'.

throughout Wallasey until the 1880s, as another convenience *provided by Providence.* The ashpit was similar to the privy midden, the contents theoretically being mixed with ash to provide 'dry conservancy.' In 1865 between 100 and 200 ashpits were being emptied monthly by the night-soil contractor in Wallasey and increased to over 1000 by 1890.

A letter to the Local Government Board in London in 1875, from Mr Fitzpatrick in Liscard vividly illustrates what, for many of the householders in the district, conditions must have been like:

> *Esk Cottage,*
> *Wallasey Road*
> *Liscard, Cheshire*
>
> *23rd September 1875*
>
> *The Secretary*
> *Local Government Board*
> *London*
>
> *Sir,*
> *I beg to call the attention of your Honourable Board to the entire absence of drainage here.*
> *While I write there are from three to four inches of water in the kitchens and back passages. The only outlet for sewage is an open drain running at the back of the house and emitting at times the most abominable stench.*
> *From the WC, which is simply a cesspool in the yard there is no drainage whatever, and the sewage leaks away the best it can. I am informed that the road is sewered to within about forty yards of this house. But the Local Board of Works and Health seem to have no power to go any further. I have spoken to my landlord, who is quite ready to drain if there were anything to drain into, but under the circumstances can do nothing. I have called the attention to the Surveyor of the Local board for the District to the matter. The Local Board have been memorialised and now I appeal to you to do something.*
> *I feel sure that if you were aware how great the nuisance is you would take immediate steps for its abatement.*
> *I am, Sir,*
> *Your Obedient Servant*
> *W. Kirkpatrick*

The water closet, the forerunner of the lavatory of today, is first mentioned in the Wallasey Health Committee minutes of September, 1859. The Surveyor, reporting on a privy and ashpit in Union St that he found to be in a *very offensive state*, suggested that the only remedy was for their complete removal and conversion into WCs. There were problems with the WC at the Board Offices in 1865 and the Surveyor was instructed *to get the water closet in the Public Office examined by some competent person from Liverpool, without delay, in order that the bad smell which issues there from may be remedied.* During the 1860s there began a drive to convert the privies into WC's. There are frequent notices given by the Surveyor, in some cases on a doctor's advice, for owners to make the conversion. The costs were not inconsiderable. In 1875 the price quoted for such a conversion was £27. 19 shillings four pence. The Wallasey Local Board was ambivalent to such work at times; perhaps this was due to pressure from landlords and the costs involved. In 1871, for instance, the Surveyor had recommended the introduction of trough water closets into the courts of Seacombe as the only means of remedying the unhealthy situation there. The Health Committee actually went on an inspection of the courts and alleys of Seacombe on 4 October 1871. However the motion proposed, to require the provision of the trough water closets, was lost by the Chairman's casting vote. Somebody must have informed the Medical Department of the Local Government Board in London about this decision. A short time later the Wallasey Board received the following letter, signed by Dr John Simon, the Chief Medical Officer:

> *Medical Department of the Local Government Board*
> *3, Parliament Street,*
> *London, SW*
>
> *11th November 1871*
>
> *Sir*
> *I am directed by the Local Government Board to call attention of the Local Board of Wallasey to the foul and unhealthy condition of some of the courts at Seacombe arising from privies and midden-steads improperly constructed and containing large accumulations of excrement and refuse. The state of the courts has already been brought under the notice of the Local Board, by Mr Radcliffe, one of the Inspectors of this Department, who, after inspecting them, communicated with the chairman of the Local Board on the subject; but the Local government Board are informed that no steps have been taken to carry out Mr Radcliffe's recommendations, and that the nuisances still remain unabated.*
> *I am directed to say that the Local Board should at once exercise the powers conferred on them by the 57th section of the Public Health act 1848 by compelling the provision of proper water closets and ashpits, and their general powers in regard to the removal of nuisances, in order to remedy the unwholesome conditions reported by Mr Radcliffe; and in this connection I am to call particular attention of the Board to the 49th section of the Sanitary Act 1866.*
> *The Local Government Board request to be informed with as little delay as possible what measures the Local Board of Wallasey decide to adopt in the matter.*
> *I am, Sir*
> *Your obedient Servant*
> *John Simon*

The 1866 Sanitary Act referred to, allowed the Home Secretary to take proceedings when a local authority failed to act and to charge the local authority for the work. Shortly after receiving this letter the Wallasey Local Board authorised the Surveyor to *provide water closets in Seacombe in default of the owner*. However, in 1873 the Health Committee was presented with a list of houses in High Seacombe where the Surveyor felt privies required

converting to WCs. The Committee resolved that such work was *not desirable* and instructed the Surveyor to ensure that the ashpits were *well looked after*.

It was only from about 1880 when there was a concerted and continuous effort to improve matters, as the Medical Officer, Dr Cragimile, reports in 1886. *It is really only in the last six years that any such conversion of privies and formation of proper ashpits, with more frequent cleansing, has been carried out on a systematic and larger scale.* Dr Craigmile must take credit for zealously pushing the Board to carry out such work. He stated in 1885 that *I think it is almost impossible to overrate the good done by clearing away rows of these foul smelling privies, not that there is any direct proof of illness as such, but that persons and especially children, habitually breathing foul air from them, get insensibly a lower vitality and fall readier to infection than would otherwise be the case.* Between 1885 and 1890, 1126 offensive privies were converted to WCs.

This improvement and modernisation was dependent on a plentiful supply of water and efficient drains and sewers. There were frequent notices served to 'drain and sewer' in the 1840s, but the general sewerage of Wallasey developed in rather a haphazard manner initially. There was resistance from local property owners who were partly liable for the costs. In answer to Robert Rawlinson's question, at the 1851 enquiry, *is there any general system of sewerage?* The Commissioners' reply was succinct *we have no general system of sewerage*. During the rest of this decade not much progress was made. There are frequent notices served 'to drain' houses but also frequent complaints about the ineffective sewers. In 1864 the Wallasey Health Committee were *satisfied that no sewer is required in the Seacombe locality at present* although the following year there was some sewering work done in Oakdale Road. Many of the arguments and delays were down to cost. The Local Board could borrow money for sewer construction from Government funds but the Board also tried to ensure that local ratepayers contributed. The Green Lane saga of 1870 illustrates such an argument between the Local Board and local residents. 14 residents of Green Lane [12 market gardeners, 1 mason and 1 timber dealer] wrote to the Local Government Board in Whitehall on 14 February 1870:

> *We, the undersigned Landowners and Residents in the Village of Wallasey, having hitherto failed to induce the Local Board of Health to take notice of our complaint beg to represent to you the deplorable state of the village known as Wood Lane and Green Lane and respectively request an inspection may be made at the same by your officer.*
> *At present the roads in question are little better than swamps; a great number of cottages are situated in them and although good drainage is quite easy and would be inexpensive to carry out, no attempt has hitherto been made to effect this desirable work.*
> *Fever has more than once originated here and has been frequently rife; fearing a return to this in the coming spring, your requisionists hope this complaint may be promptly inquired into.*

The Wallasey Board was not keen for a Government inquiry and Mr Lea, the Surveyor, was dismissive of the complaints in his reply to Whitehall.
Mr Lea reported that:

Wood Lane and Green Lane were totally unmade and that the surface is incapable of being cleansed by ordinary means. The only pool of water of an objectionable character was an area of some six superficial yards and that there was refuse of clothes washing deposited there most likely by some of the inhabitants in the immediate vicinity. The liability of the cost of drainage would rest upon the owners of the land abutting upon the lanes in question and that in the absence of the sea or a sewer being within 100 feet the Board has no power to compel the owners to make such a sewer. He concludes by stating that *the nuisance complained of is in my opinion much exaggerated and that it arises from the untidy habits of one or two only, out of an aggregate of eleven cottages. The only remedy for this, and other minor nuisances in the locality is by executing the scheme of drainage already executed to the Board at an estimated cost of £10,000.*

The Board appear to have won the argument as the Secretary of State's opinion was that the matter be left in the hands of the Wallasey Board but that the Board should *be encouraged to proceed with the large main sewer to the area as soon as local circumstances justify.* Game, set and match to the Board!

In 1874 the Medical Officer of Health reported several cases of scarlatina in Wallasey and advised that an *extension of the sewerage system in that township was much wanted.* Gradually the sewerage system was put in place. In 1875 a sewerage works was constructed in Wheatland Lane at a cost of £550. The Surveyor optimistically stated in 1879 that *the sewerage of Wallasey is rapidly drawing to a close.* It was ten years later, in his 1889 report, when the Medical Officer of Health felt happy about the drains and sewers, stating *I have no hesitation in saying that the old system of private drainage in our district has been quite revolutionised.* There were still some complaints about unpleasant sewer smells and Keeling's Sewer Gas Destructors were erected, one in Mount Road and the other in Grove Road. By 1896 the Medical Officer was even happier to report *towards the close of 1896 the council resolved to spend about £30,000 on the main sewer. This I believe to be the most important step in connection*

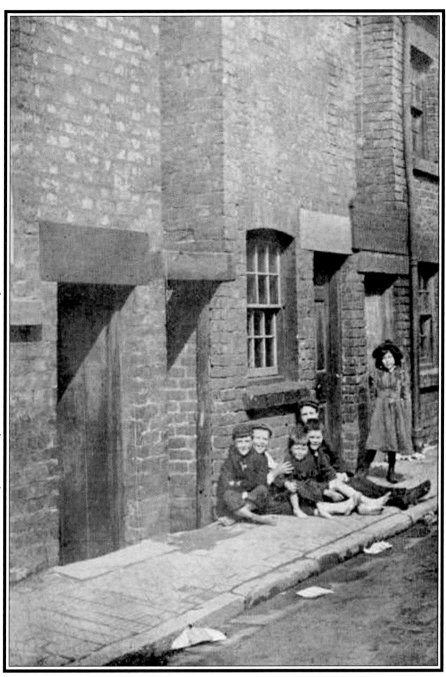

This view of the fronts of houses in Mersey Street Seacombe, with entrances to a back yard common to two houses, was taken in 1908. Although some of the children are barefooted and there is litter about, conditions here some 30 years earlier were far worse, as described in this chapter.

with the sanitary condition of the district that has been taken for the past 20 years.

Thus, by the turn of the century, Wallasey generally had a system of sewerage and drainage up to the needs of a population of 52,000 and was certainly better equipped for the twentieth century than it had been 50 years earlier. It is difficult to quantify the beneficial effect that these improvements had on the population at the time. The benefits of the investment were not seen until Edwardian times, and beyond, when the death rate from infection, particularly amongst children, finally began to fall.

NIGHT-SOILMEN

The chief obstacle to the immediate removal of decomposing refuse of towns and habitations has been the expense and annoyance of the hand labour and cartage requisite for the purpose.

Edwin Chadwick, Inquiry into the Sanitary Conditions of the Labouring Population of Great Britain – 1842

This must have been the most unpleasant job of the era! The chapter on cesspits describes the growing problem of filth, excrement and rubbish that accumulated as the population of Wallasey grew. The task of removing this fell to the scavengers and night-soilmen. The night-soilmen were so called because their job was to shovel the muck into carts and remove and deposit this elsewhere. The disturbance of the muck would fill the air with an abominable stench and so it was preferable to the populace to have this unpleasant, smelly removal done at night.

In the 1840s there was no formal system for emptying the ashpits and cesspits. In October 1845, a Mr Lewis wrote to the Wallasey Commissioners asking how he was *to proceed respecting the emptying of his ashpit and removal of the contents.* The Commissioners simply replied to him that there was *nothing in the Act of Parliament to prevent the emptying and removal of the contents of Ashes and Night-soil provided it be done between the hours of midnight and five o'clock in the morning.* With this reply it must have been tempting for Mr Lewis to simply leave things as they were rather than going out to empty his ashpit at the dead of night! The first mention of a more formal system being considered is in June 1849 when the Surveyor was instructed to *remove all filth and noxious matters which may be found, deposited or accumulated on the public highway or private streets . . . with all justifiable expedition.*

In 1851 Robert Rawlinson, on sampling the smells of Seacombe was reminded of experiencing *the tainted atmosphere in a thickly populated street of Liverpool during the labours of the night scavengers* and he could not forget *the horribly nauseating smell.* The night-soilmen were described as being *very filthy in appearance and habits.* Indeed, in Wallasey there were frequent complaints about their behaviour, including damage to property while they were going about their business. In 1872 there were complaints from residents that the night-soilmen were extorting money from parties whose ashpits they were emptying.

In 1853 the matter was discussed again and the Surveyor was authorized to employ a team of men to scavenge for filth. This was to be deposited *in situations deemed least objectionable.* This job was initially done by the Surveyor's labourers but the following year it was decided to put the removal of night-soil out to tender. The dubious honour of the first contract for the removal of night-soil went to a Mr

Joshua Dean in July 1854; he was paid £100 for 12 months. Almost immediately begins a catalogue of complaints about the final resting place of the night soil that lasts until the end of the century. Mr Dean appears to have dumped the night-soil on his field in Liscard, as manure, and there were complaints from his neighbour. The next contract went to a lady, Mrs Jemimah Taylor. She won a three year contract, from August 1855, being paid £150 for the first year, £160 for the second year and £170 for the final year. She nearly lost the contract in 1856 when she was found depositing night-soil on the shore at New Brighton. She was then required to provide depots, the site to be agreed with the Surveyor, where the night-soil would be dumped. There were obviously clashes between Mrs Taylor and the Surveyor as she complained of the *ill feeling shown towards her by him.* In 1857 there were continuing complaints about Mrs Taylor's performance and the Board decided to take over the collection of night-soil themselves and terminated her contract.

In 1860 the wages of the night-soilmen were three shillings two pence (16p) per night. In 1865 their wages were increased from 18 shillings to £1 per week.

In 1866 the Board put the night-soil removal out to contract again and Mr Thomas Monk took on the job. The contract by then was worth £400 per year. The night-soil removal seems to have run smoothly until 1872 when it was reported to the Board that *Mr Thomas Monk, the contractor for removal of night-soil, had been guilty of such negligence as to compel the Surveyor to give him notice that if the contract was not properly carried out he would recommend the Board to sue him for the penalties therein provided.*

When the night-soil contract came up for renewal in 1873 there was little interest from local contractors and the initial advertisement drew no response at all! Eventually Mr Henry Little took the contract, for £600 a year, after the Board estimated it would cost them £700 per year to revert to taking on the job themselves. At this stage about 150 ashpits a month were being emptied. The following year the Board again decided to take on the work themselves but after proposals to buy their own horses and carts, they had second thoughts and put the job out to tender again. Mr Little took the contract again, now receiving £750 per year. In 1875 the Wallasey Board were instructed by the Local Government Board that house refuse should be collected from premises at the same time. By now Mr Little had problems complying with the contract, perhaps because of this extra work. In 1876 the ashpit emptying was way behind schedule and Mr Little said this was partly *due to the loss of one of his horses and the lameness of another.* The Board was not impressed with his excuse!

Mr John Robinson took the contract in 1876. This was now worth £820 for the first year, £950 for the second and £1100 for third year. By now there was becoming increasing difficulty for the contractor to dispose of the night-soil. In

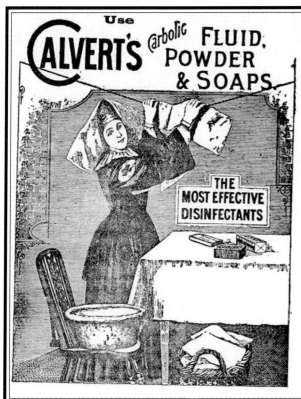

This 1892 advert for Calvert's Carbolic products includes Carbolic Disinfecting Powder which was supplied by the Wallasey Board used as a disinfectant for sprinkling into ashpits (*see this page*).

July 1877 Mr Robinson asked the Wallasey Board where he *might deposit night soil from the New Brighton district, as he did not know where to put it to be free from complaints.* The Board was not helpful and told him they could not assist in the matter. Soon afterwards there are complaints of the night-soil ending up on ground around new cottages in New Brighton and on local fields. Interestingly, when the Medical Officer was asked to look into matters he did not feel the spreading of *the night-soil superficially over fields as manure was injurious.* It still must have smelt awful!

In 1879 the contract went to Mr JR and JJ Hickson; £2760 for three years. There continued to be intermittent complaints of the contractor falling behind in his emptying of the ashpits. Mr George Fogg took the tender in 1883; £1140 for one year. Disinfection is first mentioned; the contractor was to be supplied with Calvert's Carbolic Powder (*see advert on this page*) for sprinkling into the ashpits, after emptying. Wrought iron dirt boxes cost ten shillings each at this time.

One of the Health Committee duties, in 1886, is formally stated as being responsible for arranging and regulating the removal of night-soil and to provide depots *for storage, use or destruction of all night-soil.* Mr John Robinson has another spell as contractor this year, for £900. The penalty clauses in the contract stated that:
each ashpit or receptacle should be emptied within 24 hours from receipt of notice, and in no case should exceed 72 hours or a penalty of Five shillings (25p) per day, per ashpit, would be enforced.
Mr Robinson was threatened with this penalty on several occasions.

Not only did the people of Wallasey have to put up with their own rubbish and muck. In 1887 the Board took a Mr Gracy from Birkenhead to court, and won. He was accused of depositing ashpit refuse from Birkenhead on land at the Model Farm in Wallasey. *Large quantities of the most offensive part of the refuse from Birkenhead* were carted across and dumped here. Dr Craigmile adds to the picture in his annual report of 1888 mentioning that:
It came out in evidence that Birkenhead still had a large number of these open privies and that their contents had been spread on the land creating such an intolerable smell that proceedings had to be taken to protect residents in the neighbourhood.

Mr George Fogg took the night-soil tender again in 1888 for less payment than earlier in that decade; £1980 for two years. In this year it is noted 3609 ashpits had been emptied since the beginning of the year which would equate to about 225 per week.

There was still some ingenuity in dumping night-soil, even at the end of the 1880s. There was a complaint that night-soil had been left in the enclosure of the Reformed Church of England, Martins Lane, Liscard. When it comes to night soil, it seems nowhere was sacred!

It was not until the 1890s that the problem of night-soil dumping was finally resolved. In the early 1890s the Medical Officer was still frustrated by the *vexed question* as to solving the problem. In 1895, after several years of discussion, a Refuse Destructor was opened at the bottom of Gorsey Lane, to incinerate the growing volume of rubbish. The Wallasey Council took over the collection of rubbish in 1897 when 480 dustbins were in use and emptied weekly. In this year, extolling the virtues of using dustbins, the Medical Officer was able to report that:

the noisy and offensive emptying of ashpits is done away with and a revolution in the old system is being quietly effected.

In 1900 he reiterated his like of dustbins:

this method does away with the old and bad method of wheeling out the contents of ashpits [often foul and decomposing] to be emptied on the road and left till the cart comes round to remove them. It also does away with the noise and disturbance of the barrows and shovelling - formerly a great annoyance to householders.

Although the problems of collection were thus resolved the habits of some of the population proved difficult to change and people were obviously reluctant to use the new fangled dustbins, as the Medical Officer's rather pessimistically reports in 1906:

I must confess that I am often surprised to see great heaps of night-soil lying in some of our roads occupied by good houses waiting till the carts come round to collect it. It is no wonder that in poor localities the tenants or landlords do not go to the expense – trifling as it is – of providing bins, where ashpits are already in existence; but it is a matter of astonishment that the tenants of large houses should put up year after year with the old ash-pits harbouring all sorts of refuse for six weeks or more, when a weekly collection by means of the bins is offered by the Council. Unless compulsory powers are got to adopt the bin system, it appears the old system of ash-pits will still linger for a long time.

THE DEAD HOUSE

He'd make a lovely corpse.

Charles Dickens, Martin Chuzzlewhit

In its early days the primary use of the Dead House, or mortuary, seems to have been for the reception of drowned corpses. Mr Thomas Westcott, in his *Memoirs of Wallasey*, recalls that the only mortuary in the parish in the 1850s was in an old cottage at the back of the *Black Horse* yard. It was apparently not unusual for the innkeeper to receive the order *to make room for a drowned man*. Mr Westcott remembers this order being given many times and the sleepless nights that the family had on this account. He tells an amusing story of one such drowned sailor who was put in the stable beside the old cottage. Alarm was caused when noises were heard from the stable and on further investigation the dead man had come to life. He was dead when put in the stable – dead drunk!. Mr Westcott hastens

to add that the man was from Birkenhead, not Wallasey.

The want of a proper Dead House was first raised by the Wallasey Board in July 1859, after complaints from local hotels and public houses about the unsatisfactory arrangements. The Board applied to The Secretary of State for the Home Department for permission to spend ratepayers money on providing such a facility for the district.

Liverpool
30th July 1859

Sir,
I am directed by the Wallasey Board of Health to request the favour of your opinion on the following point. The District of the Local Board is bounded on the North and East by the Irish Sea and the River Mersey, on the Strand of which bodies of persons drowned are frequently washed, left by the receding tide.

When found they are taken to the nearest Hotel or Public House where they remain until an Inquest is held and an order made for their internment.

A delay of two or three days sometimes takes place before such internment.

It is highly objectionable to the Proprietors of the Houses referred to and their visitors that the corpses should be taken there, but at present there is no alternative.

By the Public Health Act of 1848 Local Boards are empowered 'for the purpose of preventing the manifold evils occasioned by the retention of the dead in the dwellings of the poor to provide premises for the internment of corpses until burial.'

The question is whether the Wallasey Local Board would be justified in providing out of the General District Rates a building or room or even two or three buildings or rooms in convenient parts of the District for reception of corpses under the circumstances mentioned.

I have the honour to be,
Sir,
Your most obedient humble servant,
TK Hassle
The Clerk to the Local Board

This was sanctioned and in August the matter was discussed with the coroner, with a view to finding a suitable site. However, the following month the Health Committee was having difficulty in finding a convenient site for 'such houses' and put the matter aside. Despite the apparent urgency of the situation there is then no further mention of the Dead House for a further two years.

The Board was reminded of the situation in June 1861 when they received a memorial from certain inhabitants of New Brighton and elsewhere. The Board's attention was drawn to *the great want of a Dead House in the Parish for the reception of Dead Bodies cast ashore*. The memorialists suggested that a suitable site might be the old Lifeboat House at the Magazines *as a convenient and central location*. The Board applied to the Mersey Docks and Harbour Board, who owned the premises, but the Harbour Board declined to let for use as a Dead House.

The Board responded by resolving to put up iron posts and a rail at Seacombe *to prevent accidents caused by the rapid descent from Victoria Road.* They also resolved to repair some railings at the slip at Seacombe. Presumably they were hoping such measures would reduce the number of drownings caused by such accidents, and lessen the need for the Dead House. Perhaps these measures helped as it was another four years until the Dead House was finally established. There is a brief note in the Board minutes in September 1865 to say that a Dead House had been established at the Old Boat House at the Magazines, for a rent of £6 per annum.

The old habits of using the nearest hotel seem to have persevered, as the Board discussed in September 1869.

> *29th September 1869*
> *While the Board paid a rental for permission to use one of the Old Lifeboat Houses at the Magazines a Dead House, and has filled up the same for that purpose, the Sergeant of Police, on Saturday last, persisted in placing the dead body of a person drowned at New Brighton in the stables behind the* Royal Ferry Hotel *and in close proximity to several dwellings.*

A complaint was sent to the Chief Constable, *in order to prevent a repetition of the evil complained of.* The Chief Constable looked into the matter and reported that the Sergeant had taken the body to the hotel:
in the hope that the medical man sent for might have been able to resuscitate him and under such circumstance it would have been improper to convey him to the Dead House.
Unfortunately, in this case, unlike the earlier case reported by Mr Westcott it appears the unfortunate person was dead and not 'dead drunk'.

In 1870 a bearing barrow for carrying dead was provided for Seacombe Ferry, from one of the two kept at the Dead House at the Magazines. In 1871 the Mersey Docks and Harbour Board offered to sell the Old Lifeboat House to the Board, as repairs were necessary. The Board decided to undertake the repairs themselves, and continued renting the premises.

The premises served for the rest of the 1870s. In September 1880 there was a proposal to site a mortuary, as it was now called, at Seacombe Ferry. The building needed was to be 16 feet long, 12 feet wide and 10 feet 6 inches wide at an estimated cost of £40.

The Dead House at the Magazines was still in use in 1887. The owner was a Mr Melling and he did give notice to the Board asking that the premises *be given up on the 1st July next, and the doors of the same to be restored to their original condition.* Mr Melling, however, relented when the Board offered to increase the rent from £6 to £9 per year.

POLLUTION
The River Mersey

> *The river is within us, the sea is all about us.*
>
> TS Eliot, *Four Quartets,* '*Dry Salvages*'

The River Mersey's influence on the health of Wallasey was appreciated during the reign of Victoria, although it was not until King Edward's reign that these influences were more fully recognised. It is perhaps understandable that the efforts of the Wallasey Local Board were directed towards creating sewers, removing filth and rubbish from streets and houses and disinfecting and isolating cases of fever rather than tackling river pollution. The river was a convenient and free outlet for sewage and rubbish.

The Mersey played an integral part of Wallasey life in the nineteenth century. In the early part of the century it provided a livelihood; the rural population included fishermen, whose lives were often in the hands of the elements. As Wallasey began to develop as a residential district, so the ferries developed, with increasing traffic between Wallasey and Liverpool. In 1823 steam packets were plying between Seacombe and Liverpool every hour. By 1876 there were one and three quarter million passengers using the Seacombe ferry annually. As New Brighton developed as a resort, so increasing numbers of day trippers would arrive from Liverpool and beyond. From further afield came canal boats, plying their trade. There was also contact with merchant and passenger ships from around the world.

Robert Rawlinson, in his sanitary report on Poulton-cum-Seacombe of 1851, vividly describes both the attractions and drawbacks of Wallasey's location on the river.
The attractions – *The whole line of shore from Seacombe Ferry round to the Leasowe embankment consists of favourable site for building, from which a panoramic view of an unrivalled character may be obtained. The waters of the Mersey bear much of the commerce of the world; vessels of every size, and from every clime, visit the port. Liverpool, with its six miles of river wall and docks, its forest of masts, its warehouses, towers, spires and domes, is presented to the view of the inhabitants of Seacombe; and at night hundreds of lamps light up the quays and the town, affording to the spectator on the Cheshire shore all the effect of a jubilant illumination. The coloured lamps indicating the several dock entrances give the character of a fete, and the moving lights in the vessels and steamers impart animation to the scene.*

In the same report is the less savoury side of being on the river bank. A Mr Banner, at the Rawlinson Inquiry on 31 July 1851, at *Parry's Hotel,* Seacombe, pointed out of the window to show cesspool matter spread out on the beach below. Paradoxically, as sewers and drains improved during

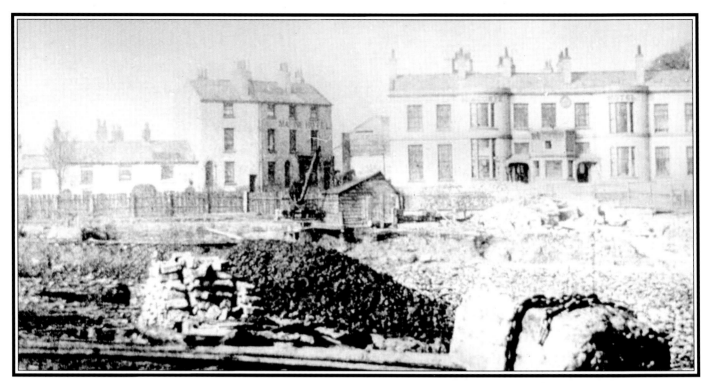

This view of Seacombe Ferry, taken c.1876, shows work has started on rebuilding the ferry. The Seacombe Ferry Hotel to the right, was was once run by Thomas Parry and is the 1850s Parry's Hotel mentioned in this chapter. Marine Hotel is to the left.

the last quarter of the century, pollution of the river with sewage actually worsened. In 1880 Miss Smith of New Brighton complained to the Health Committee about sewer outlets on the shore between Egremont Ferry and the Magazines. These were emptying above the low water mark, so when the tide was out one can imagine the consequence! The cost of remedying such problems must have made it difficult for people to decide whether it was worth putting up with the unpleasantness. In this case the Surveyor estimated the cost of moving the outlets below the low water mark to be £2,200, the cost to be borne by the various owners whose properties adjoined the shore.

Being near the estuary of the Mersey, Wallasey would have received a concentration of flotsam, jetsam and things more unpleasant from the populations and factories up-river. In 1855 there were complaints that the Local Board was not removing dead dogs, cats and other animals left on the shore by the tide. In 1859 the Board resolved that *all dead dogs found on the shore should be immediately buried.* The Surveyor, in 1866, reports that 18 dead dogs a week were being washed ashore, allegedly thrown into the river by the Liverpool police! Not many miles upstream, at Warrington in 1876, the Mersey was described as *Black as ink at most times, and most offensive in smells.* Nationally the subject of river pollution was widely debated in the last quarter of the century, but despite various acts and boards being set up, such pollution steadily worsened. The Mersey and Irwell Joint Committee, set up in 1891, did have some success in reducing pollution of the Mersey upstream of Wallasey.

It was not only dead animals that one was likely to encounter on a stroll along the river bank throughout this period. One was quite likely to come across human bodies, the victims

of drowning. Looking at the Wallasey Parish Register, covering 1574 until 1812, there are drownings reported most years from the 1760s. These make poignant reading, as many seem to have met a watery end without being eventually missed or recognised eg.

1812	
March 16	A man and a male child, unknown, found drowned
April 16	A boy, unknown, found drowned
April 28	A woman, unknown, found drowned
April 30	A sergeant and private, unknown, found drowned
May 11	John Tate, found drowned in the Mersey in the township of Seacombe (a native of Down, Ireland)

Drownings continue at a similar rate throughout the century and in his annual reports, from 1885, Dr Craigmile comments on the effect that these drowning accidents had in raising the overall death rate for Wallasey. He states that the accidents happened partly from bathing accidents and partly from seamen and others falling off the dock or river walls. It appears bathing accidents were common. As early as 1866 Dr Bell wrote to the Local Board pointing out the *dangers of allowing persons to bathe so near to the Fort at New Brighton.* The Board then appointed designated swimming areas defined by posts as 'Ladies' Bathing Ground' and 'Gentlemen's Bathing Ground'. Illustrative figures, from the Medical Officer's Reports, show that between 1885 and 1890 there were 53 drownings – 19 residents of Wallasey and 34 non residents.

The consequences of such fertile pollution meant that the

river must have been an extraordinary bacterial breeding ground of water borne organisms such as typhoid and 'stomach bugs' which could be picked up by people swimming in the river, or children playing on the shore. Although the general dangers of raw sewage in promoting 'fever' on the shore were recognised at the Rawlinson enquiry in 1851, it is not until after 1900 that there begins to be mention of the possible dangers of consuming the fruits of the Mersey. In 1908 Dr Barlow, the Medical Officer of Health, warns of the dangers of eating shellfish taken from the Mersey:

I have often noticed people gathering mussels from the mussel beds on the Egremont shore and at New Brighton. I desire to draw public attention to the danger of eating shellfish from such an obviously polluted source as the River Mersey, receiving as it does, the crude sewage of approximately one million people. Notices prohibiting the gathering of these fish are exhibited in various places, but no notice is taken of them.

Factors such as the eating of shellfish, perhaps as a staple diet, may help explain the high level of typhoid in Wallasey in the latter part of the century, which so tried Dr Craigmile.

The River Mersey also had an indirect effect on the health of Wallasey residents as a means of communication, by ferry, with Liverpool. Both Dr Craigmile and Dr Barlow, the Wallasey Medical Officers of Health, when investigating the causes of outbreaks of diseases such as smallpox, frequently attributed the source to people who had contracted the infection while working in Liverpool. In his annual report of 1887 Dr Craigimile states that *in an urban district like ours we are yet in such close and constant communication with the cities of Liverpool and Birkenhead that nearly all epidemics prevailing in these centres of population are speedily imported into our own locality.*

The variety of shipping using the Mersey led to some unusual matters for Wallasey Health Committee to deal with. In April 1874 they had to write to the Admiralty asking for the removal of a gunpowder boat that was moored just offshore of Liscard Manor House. The Admiralty was informed that the gunpowder boat was *moored in an unsafe and unsuitable position.*

Factories

> *I am always conscious of an uncomfortable sensation now and then when the wind is blowing in the east.*
>
> **Charles Dickens, Bleak House**

There were worries and complaints about the effect of local industry on health, especially as industry developed in the Seacombe area from the 1830s. There were limekilns, giving the name to Limekiln Lane. In 1841 there were already copper works, smelt works, phospho-guano works, a foundry and a starch and vitriol works at Seacombe. Over

the next two decades a pottery, sugar works and cement works were also in this area.

There were complaints about most of these establishments! In 1847 there were complaints from Seacombe residents about smoke nuisance from a newly erected foundry. The Surveyor found the complaint was well grounded and the owners were instructed to raise the chimney, to reduce the smoke problem. In 1856 the inhabitants of Wheatland Lane were disturbed by *an immense quantity of black smoke emitted from the chimneys of the Potteries and the Works adjoining.* Medical opinion on factory pollution matters was called upon, before the appointment of a Medical Officer of Health. In 1862 Dr Byerley and Dr Law investigated complaints about the Artificial Manure Manufacturing Factory of Messrs Dixon and Co, Seacombe, following complaints about the *nauseous and injurious effects of the gas emanating from such works.* The doctors reported that *they found a certain quantity of Sulphurous Acid Gas which they believed was so diluted by the atmosphere as to be not materially injurious to the health of the inhabitants in the vicinity.* Despite this reassurance the Health Committee decided to take proceedings against Messrs Dixon and Co, only to find that as the factory had been established for over six months that the Public Health Act did not apply. The complainants were advised all that they could do was to take out private proceedings. The inhabitants of Seacombe did not fare any better when raising concerns about the recently erected Vitriol Works in 1872. The Vitriol Works manufactured hydrochloric acid, used, amongst other things, in the manufacture of soap. The manufacture of hydrochloric acid could lead to the acid escaping into the local atmosphere, and the sulphurated hydrogen that escaped smelt of rotten eggs. Mr Alfred Fletcher, the Government Inspector of Alkali Works, was asked to inspect the works and he had few concerns for the local population. He concluded his report as follows: *In conclusion I would say that in a district abounding with trees a vitriol works would do damage . . . but in such a district as the one where the works is placed, which is partly of a manufacturing character, there need be no fear of damage to animal or vegetable health if due care is excercised – a carelessly conducted vitriol works is a nuisance anywhere.* Perhaps he was right, as there were no further complaints made about the Vitriol Works to the Health Committee.

Seacombe was not the only area affected by obnoxious smoke and fumes. In 1863 there were numerous complaints about smoke from the Steam Chimney at Mr Ellis Davis's Mill in Liscard. The police were called to help with the proceedings against Mr Davis and he was fined five pounds. The Smoke Act of 1853 was used in such cases, stating that a fine could be imposed *if any person shall carry on a trade or business which shall occasion any noxious or offensive effluvia or otherwise annoy the neighbourhood or inhabitants.*

In the 1880s the nuisance from smoke seems to have mainly come from brick kilns. In 1880 Mr Spedding, at Comely

Bank, Seacombe, was on several occasions reported for causing *dense volumes of black smoke to issue from a brick kiln, on his premises.* He does not seem to have taken much notice of the complaints until 1882 when the Medical Officer issued a medical certificate stating that the burning of bricks in open kilns *was a nuisance injurious to the health of the inhabitants of Brighton Street, Sandon Terrace and Falkland Road.* Legal proceedings were then taken against Mr Spedding. Other complaints at this time, on possible health grounds were made against fish gut cleaning and blood drying premises in Seacombe, and about fumes from Messrs Lyons Copper Works.

With the closure of many of the businesses, such as the Seacombe Pottery and Foundry in the early 1870s the air pollution from these larger factories would have lessened. However, as Seacombe and Poulton residents of today know, there are still some days, at the end of the twentieth century, when similar smells and smoke drift across the locality.

ANIMALS

Of sheep, pigs, cows, camels and giraffes

At the beginning of the 19th century, when the three townships of Wallasey had a mainly agricultural population of about 700 people, one would expect to see farm animals as part of the rustic scene. As Wallasey grew and became urbanised the animals were not left to the 'countryside' but became a part of urban life and were kept in shippons and pigsties amongst the houses, to the continued annoyance of neighbours, the medical men and the Health Committee. Until the last decade of the century there were frequent complaints about the proximity of animals; pigs seem to have been the main cause of complaint, although cows and sheep were also much in evidence. Throughout the last half of the century there must have been a mixture of animals and humanity that we town dwellers would have difficulty with now. There would have been stables, pigsties, shippons and slaughterhouses amongst the houses and cows, pigs, chickens and sheep on the street.

As early as 1845 there were complaints about pigsties, so at this time there was already a clash between urban and rural cultures. At this time the complaint had to have the support of six inhabitant ratepayers to be entertained by the Commissioners. In the poorer districts, with fewer ratepayers, one would have been fairly powerless to complain and would have no choice but to live with the neighbours' animals. Some pigsties were removed in the 1850s but as often as not the complaints were not upheld and the complainant told that there was no problem, on the evidence of a single visit from the Surveyor. In March 1862 there was a complaint about stables and a shippon below a Mr Birch's house. The Surveyor found *nothing more objectionable than the smell usually found in stables and shippons and could not even perceive that smell when in Mr Birch's house.* People were sometimes driven to taking

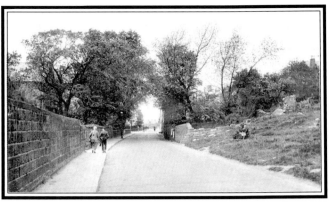

A pinfold, as mentioned in this chapter, is derived from an Anglo Saxon word for enclosure or 'pound'. Stray cattle or animals would be held there by the local authority until payment of rent or 'poundage'. The walls of the last one in Wallasey are pictured on the right in Breck Road.

their own action. Mr Stanley Sutton did so in 1870. He ordered his men to pull down a pinfold (*see photo on this page*) after complaints from his tenants that the building was *offensive from the pigs, donkeys and other animals detained therein and that their dung and droppings were allowed to remain and decompose on the ground.* Unfortunately for Mr Sutton it transpired that the pinfold was owned by the Local Board and they were not pleased. When the matter came before the Health Committee there was no debate about the possible health hazard caused by such a place and Mr Sutton contritely offered to re-erect the pinfold. The complaints about pigsties continued throughout this period. In September 1877 pigs were removed from behind the Wallasey Dispensary following a complaint by Mr W Broome, the Dispensary's Honorary Secretary and Treasurer. There were still complaints about pigsties in New Brighton in the 1880s.

There seems to have been more tolerance of cows, perhaps they were perceived as more useful or less smelly! There was no objection to cows being kept in Union Street in the 1870s. Asses were less well tolerated. In 1874 the Medical Officer inspected stables and yards in St Albans Road, where asses were kept. He found the stable in *so filthy a state as to be injurious to health.* In 1884 the Medical Officer strongly condemned the practice of keeping asses at the rear of dwelling houses.

The Medical Officer was frequently involved, with the Surveyor, in seeing whether these complaints gave rise to health risks. Surely the strangest visit they made was in June 1878, when asked to investigate smells from a menagerie at West Bank House in Egerton Street, New Brighton. Their findings were as follows:

The house recently erected by Mr Redmayne was large, commodious and well ventilated and at the time of the visit contained two camels, from which the very slightest odour emanated; less than could be perceived in the majority of stables. In the old stables they found six giraffes but could detect no smell from them likely to be injurious or at all answering the description of that complained about. On

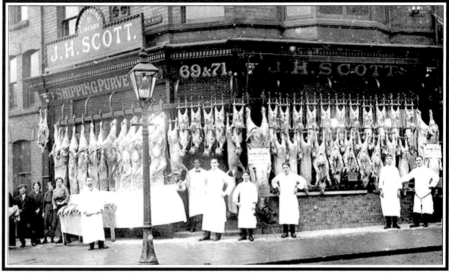

JH Scott's butcher's shop at 69–71 Victoria Road Seacombe. A few years after this photo was taken *c.*1908, the Medical Officer of Health would probably have condemned this display.

further enquiry they found that some time ago, on a Sunday, a giraffe died and Mr Redmayne admitted that it was not entirely removed for some days. The Medical Officer was of the opinion that, with proper care and attention, no nuisance whatever need be apprehended from the keeping of the Animals. Before leaving they called on Mrs Barry and satisfied her that the place should be well watched to prevent a recurrence of what had been complained about.

Part of the resistance to removing animals from the district was their use as a ready, and easy, source of both income and food. There was certainly much slaughtering of animals in the district throughout this time. Technically one had to apply for a licence to slaughter animals from the Local Board, but there was much unlicensed slaughtering. The earliest application for a licence, in the Commissioners records, is in 1849 when John Gates, a Seacombe butcher, applied for a licence to slaughter cattle at the Old Barn in Wheatland Lane. Mr Leicester's slaughterhouse in Liscard features a number of times, with repeated complaints from his neighbours about his activities, which included the boiling of bones and in 1873 a complaint that Mr Leicester made a practice of throwing blood and offal into his midden. Proceedings were taken against him by the Local Board as

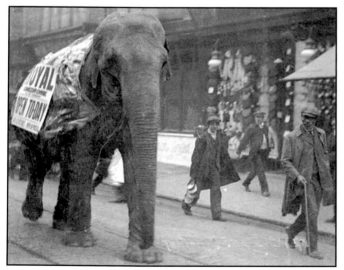

This New Brighton Tower Zoo elephant, with its keeper on the right, is seen advertising the *Royal Cinema,* Seacombe in 1914. This was not one of the zoo animals kept by Mr Redmayne which neighbours complained about in 1878!

he had been repeatedly warned on previous occasions. There were proposals for public abattoirs in 1884 but these were rejected on cost grounds. Slaughtering in unlicensed premises was still being reported in New Brighton in 1889. By 1908 there were still 12,064 animals slaughtered in seven slaughter houses in Wallasey; 87,624 animals were slaughtered at the Wallasey and Alfred Lairage at the docks.

Towards the end of the century pig keeping seems to have diminished, partly due to cheap bacon imports from America. In 1889 the sanitary sub-inspector spent much of his time at the docks examining American imports. Cows were still kept and one of the Medical Officer's duties at the end of the century, was inspecting premises from which milk was supplied. It had become clear by this time that milk was a common source of infections such as food poisoning and tuberculosis. In 1908 the Medical officer was finding cowsheds that were *very old and dark and ill ventilated and conditions were not proper for the protection of milk against infection or contamination.*

Wallasey was fairly typical of the rest of the country, with its exposure to animals, alive and dead, at this time. As elsewhere it is difficult to quantify the effect on health but the closeness to animals, in cramped conditions, and the generation of manure and dung, must have been a fertile breeding ground for bacteria. The smells and noise generated must have been unpleasant, judging by the number of complaints the Health Committee received. The output from the slaughterhouse was probably equally harmful to health; nationally, in 1862, the Privy Council estimated that one fifth of butchers meat was 'considerably diseased.' The Wallasey Medical Officer of Health and the sanitary inspectors were involved in food inspection from the time of the first Medical Officer's appointment in 1873. A variety of foodstuffs were condemned. In 1889 these included four rabbits and 234 haddocks! It was really only towards the end of the period that is being discussed, 1890 to 1910, that a fuller appreciation was reached by the Medical Officer, and the Sanitary Department, of the necessity for strict controls on both live and dead animals in the district to protect Wallasey's health.

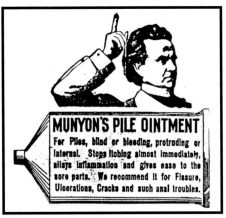

MUNYON'S PILE OINTMENT

For Piles, blind or bleeding, protruding or internal. Stops itching almost immediately, allays inflammation and gives ease to the sore parts. We recommend it for Fissure, Ulcerations, Cracks and such anal troubles.

Two of Dr Crippen's 'Quack' medicine companies (*see this page*).
Above: An advert for Munyon's Pile Ointment with Professor Munyon and raised finger.
Below: A 1902 Druet's advert from *Pearson's* magazine.

PUBLISHED IN THE INTERESTS OF THE DEAF.

Few people realise the magnitude of the work undertaken by the late Dr. Drouet in the interests of those who suffer from defective hearing and diseases of the ear. Besides creating large establishments in London, Paris, and Brussels, where aural ailments are treated by the Drouet method, he also founded a medical magazine, "The Journal for the Deaf," intended solely for the benefit of those who suffer from these afflictions. This publication contains in each issue valuable information on the care of the ears, and expressions of opinion by various authorities on the curability of deafness. Interesting instances of the cure of deafness in all its forms are also given each month in the form of a "Supplement" which contains the monthly records of the Drouet Institute. A free copy of the "Journal" and "Supplement" can be obtained by addressing the Secretary, Drouet Institute, 72, Regent's Park Road, London, N.W. With the "Journal" is always enclosed a Report Form which enables anyone to receive free advice by correspondence as to the treatment of the ear, nose, and throat. Personal consultations with the medical staff of the Drouet Institute have been arranged for every week-day between the hours of 2 and 4.

Quack Medicine

Quack Medicine was one of the great frauds in Victorian and Edwardian times. By the end of the 19th Century Americans were spending $75 million a year on patent or quack remedies and they were also popular this side of the Atlantic.

Their promises offered in advertisements were often outrageous and imposible. The reason they were so popular was that they were aimed mainly at the poor and uneducated who were unable to afford the high costs of doctors' fees, were more gullable and offered them a chance of being cured at a comparitively reasonable cost.

Many of these so called 'cures' contained large amounts of opiates, narcotics or alcohol. They ranged from powerful and dangerous heart depressants to insidious liver stimulants and often created an addiction that would need to be fed. One of these, **Peruna's Catarrh Cure**, contained 28% alcohol and resulted in a condition known as 'Peruna's jug'.

An American homoeopathic doctor, who was to become one of the 20th century's most infamous murderers – Dr Crippen, could not make a living out of homoeopathy so turned to 'Quack Medicine'. In 1894 he joined Professor Munyon, one of America's most successful Patent Medicine Kings. Their advertising included a picture of Munyon with his arm raised and index finger pointing upwards which proved to be a ribald joke with one of his remedies – **Munyons Pile Cure** (*see advert on this page*).

Dr Crippen was sent to open a London branch in 1897 where he continued to promote Munyon's Patent Medicines. He left Munyon's employment and in 1901 became a 'Consultant Physician' for the **Drouet Institute for the Deaf**. Luxurious offices were opened first at 72 Regents Park Road then at Marble Arch for this French swindle. This was a very plausible scam as they issued a medical magazine *The Journal for the Deaf* which contained information on the care of the ears. A monthly supplement on successes of the Drouet Institute was also published and both could be obtained free of charge. Inside the journal was a Report Form which could be completed and free advice given on the treatment of the ear, nose and throat. Personal consultations were offered but in practice not encouraged. A diagnosis would be made by Crippen and one of several standard letters would be returned to the sender with a diagnosis using such medical terms as 'Post Otorrhea and Tinnitus' or 'Rhinitis Chronica Rhino,

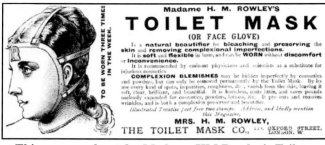

Madame H. M. ROWLEY'S

TOILET MASK

(OR FACE GLOVE)

Is a natural beautifier for bleaching and preserving the skin and removing complexional imperfections. It is soft and flexible in form, and can be WORN without discomfort or inconvenience.

It is recommended by eminent physicians and scientists as a substitute for injurious cosmetics.

COMPLEXION BLEMISHES may be hidden imperfectly by cosmetics and powders, but can only be removed permanently by the Toilet Mask. By its use every kind of spots, impurities, roughness, &c., vanish from the skin, leaving it soft, clear, brilliant, and beautiful. It is harmless, costs little, and saves pounds uselessly expended for cosmetics, powders, lotions, &c. It prevents and removes wrinkles, and is both a complexion preserver and beautifier.

Illustrated Treatise post free two stamps. Address, and kindly mention this Magazine.

MRS. H. M. ROWLEY,

THE TOILET MASK CO., 125, OXFORD STREET, LONDON, W.

This was an advert for Madame HM Rowley's Toilet Mask in an 1899 edition of *Windsor Magazine*. It claimed to remove every kind of spot and even wrinkles!

Pharyngitis, Eustachian Salpingitis', and prescribed the anti-catarrhal plasters or gargle plus nasal spray plus anti-catarrhal powders, as the case might be.

After several cases of bad publicity, Drouets downfall came following the death of a Staffordshire Locksmith who had been under treatment from the institute, using Drouet's Plasters. At the inquest a Dr Percival told the jury that this treatment using Drouet's plasters was quite useless.

Drouet's did not long survive this adverse publicity but Crippen actually profited from its misfortune as he was able to acquire Drouet's assets very reasonably, remarketing their products under his **Aural Remedies Company** label. Those replying to the Aural Remedies advertisements would receive a copy of a fake *Otological Gazette* together with an analytical form which they completed and returned to HH Crippen MD (USA) at *Craven House* Kingsway London. The treatment, which cost one guinea (£1.05), claimed that

No matter how many disappointments . . . no matter how severe, obstinate or chronic the form of deafness . . . this method has made it possible for patients to effect a positive and permanent cure by treating themselves in their own home.

However, if no reply was received a second letter would be sent out claiming they had just received a letter from a grateful client who had been entirely cured by their product having been deaf for 58 years! Also, they could take advantage of a half-price offer of ten shillings six pence (52.5p) for the 'full and complete outfit' and if they were then fully satisfied they could send the other ten shillings six pence! [Quack medicine at its best – or worst].

Dr Crippen gave a 'Medical Lecture' at the Assembly Rooms Albion Street New Brighton in 1907. It is not clear what he was lecturing about – but was probably concerned with quack medicine.

One of the more outrageous claims must have been from **Dr James W Kidd** of Fort Wayne Indiana USA whose advert on this page, taken from a *Royal* magazine of 1903, is headed **ALL DISEASES CURED.** Then he states he has letters from 70,000 satisfied customers! He goes on to list some of the cases he has cured that other doctors pronounced incurable but then contradicts himself by stating that *I have no speciality. Neither do I treat all diseases.* He then reveals his secret – which can be tried free of charge

initially but then probably convinces the 'patient' to continue with the treatment – at a cost.

For the Victorian lady with 'complexion blemishes' the answer was **Madame HM Rowley's Toilet Mask** (*see advert on this page*). The Toilet Mask (or face glove), which was to be worn three times a week, *is a natural beautifier for bleaching* [it was the fashion then to have white skin] *and preserving the skin and removing complexional imperfections.* The advertisements goes on to mention that *it is recommended* [the face mask] *by eminent physicians*

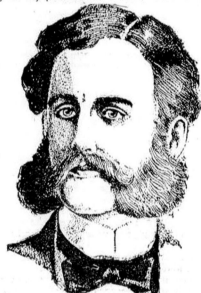

ALL DISEASES CURED.

Are you sick? Do you want to get well? If so this offer is of vital importance to you. I can show you the way to get well. It is the way that I have proven successful in thousands of cases. As I sit writing, I can see files which contain letters from seventy thousand satisfied and grateful patients who have proven the value of my treatment by actual trial. If you could read a few of these letters telling of miraculous cures after years of suffering I would need no further argument to convince you of my ability. I have passed the experimental stage. I know what I can do. No matter what your disease. I have cured many cases of Consumption, Bright's Disease, Locomotor Ataxia, and Partial Paralysis, that other doctors pronounced incurable. No matter how many doctors or patent medicines you have tried. The majority of my patients had tried all these in vain before

DR. JAMES W. KIDD.

they came to me. I CAN CURE YOU. This is a strong statement, but I am willing to show my faith in my own ability. I WILL SEND YOU A FREE TREATMENT. You can be the judge. If you are satisfied purchase further treatment if you need it. If you don't need it, recommend me to your friends. I feel sure of my pay in either case because I know what my treatment will do.

I have no speciality. Neither do I treat all diseases. Some require the bedside attention of a surgeon. If your case does I will tell you so, and the information will not cost you anything. But do not hesitate to write because someone has told you that your disease is incurable. Every organ of the body is a perfect machine and will work perfectly if it is supplied with the proper force from the nerves, and sufficient nourishment from the blood. I have learned how to supply this nerve force and blood nourishment. This is the secret of my success. This is why I can cure where others fail.

I have associated with me four of the most eminent specialists in America. Tell us all about your case. No matter what your ailment, your correspondence will be considered entirely confidential. We will make a careful examination of it. The free treatment will be prepared and sent you by mail postage paid. It only costs you a stamp. I can use no stronger argument to convince you of my ability to cure you than this. You have everything to gain, nothing to lose. Write to-day. Address my private office as follows:—Dr. JAMES W. KIDD, 430, Baltes Block, Fort Wayne, Indiana, U.S.A.

This advert was taken from a *Royal* magazine of 1903 – (*see this page*).

45

MORTIMER'S RHEUMATIC OIL.

POSSESSED OF MOST POWERFUL VIRTUES,

AND PRODUCED FROM AN ARTICLE HITHERTO UNKNOWN TO SCIENCE

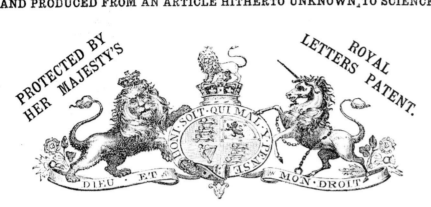

PROTECTED BY HER MAJESTY'S

ROYAL LETTERS PATENT.

For Rheumatism, Sciatica, Neuralgia, Lumbago, Bronchitis, Affections of the Chest and Throat, Croup, Cramps, Numbness of the Limbs, Coldness of the Feet, &c., also Sprains.

THE FIRST APPLICATION INVARIABLY GIVES IMMEDIATE RELIEF.

IT RECOMMENDS ITSELF.

SOLE MANUFACTURER—

J. L. MORTIMER, SEACOMBE, ENGLAND

Price 2s. 9d. per Bottle, Post Free, which includes the Government Stamp.

Telegraphic Address—"MORTIMER," SEACOMBE.

---

and scientists as a substitute for injurious cosmetics. It does not mention who these are but goes on to claim *by its use every kind of spots, impurities, roughness, etc., vanish from the skin, leaving it soft, clear, brilliant, and beautiful. It is harmless, costs little and saves pounds uselessly expended for cosmetics, powders, lotions etc*. However, if the lady is not yet convinced, the following statement would surely do the trick: *It prevents and removes wrinkles, and is both a complexion preserver and beautifier.*

Condy's Fluid (*see advert on page 30*) was advertised in a 1911 edition of the *British Medical Journal*. Its recommended uses were varied: *An antiseptic mouth wash and gargle, cleansing the throat and fauces, purifying the teeth and sweetening the breath; bracing the ulvula and fortifying the voice; purifying water for drinking and renovating filters; the deodorant for post-mortems and dissections; an injection in gonorrhoea etc.*

Three **Homocea** products were advertised in the *Illustrated Sporting and Dramatic News* of 1897 (*see this page*). The products were produced at their Homocea Works in Birkenhead and included *an unequalled remedy for burns, croup, neuralgia, ringworm, toothache and simply*

THE . . . .

JUBILEE TRIPLETS

Do not ask the Royal Bounty, but the patronage of the public, for

WE ALL - -
TOUCH THE

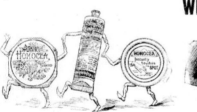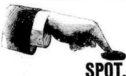

SPOT.

HOMOCEA

Unequalled as a remedy for **Burns, Bruises, Cuts, Sores,** or **Wounds. Simply wonderful in Piles,** and **Ringworm** ceases to be when Homocea is used. Invaluable in **Croup, Colds in the Head, Neuralgia, Toothache, etc., etc.**

Price, 1s. 1½d. and 2s. 9d. per box.

HOMOCEA
SOAP

The Perfection of Purity. A perfect Soap for all with Tender Skins. Makes a soft velvety lather. Is Emollient and Antiseptic. The finest and best Soap ever made. Softens the hardest water.

Price. 4d., 9d., and 1s. per Tablet.

small cake may be had free at 98, Strand, London, W.C.

HOMOCEA EMBROCATION
(Strong Homocea),
Absolutely the best thing of its kind in the World.

Put up in Collapsible Tubes, price 7½d. and 1/1½ per tube, by all dealers, and from the London Depot, 98, Strand.

All the above free by post for value in stamps from—

The HOMOCEA WORKS, BIRKENHEAD.

TRY IT IN YOUR BATH.

SCRUBB'S
CLOUDY AMMONIA.

A MARVELLOUS PREPARATION.

Refreshing as a Turkish Bath.
Invaluable for Toilet Purposes.
Splendid Cleansing Preparation for the Hair.
Removes Stains and Grease Spots from Clothing.
Allays the Irritation caused by Mosquito Bites.
Invigorating in Hot Climates.
Restores the Colour to Carpets.
Cleans Plate and Jewellery.
Softens Hard Water.
So Vivifying after Football, Motoring and other Sports.

"MAKES HOME, SWEET HOME IN DEED."

Scrubbs Cloudy Ammonia advert of the 1890s

IN THESE DAYS OF HIGH PRESSURE

when the incessant grind necessary for a decent existence is severe enough to knock vital sparks out of the constitutions of the best of us, who shall deny that they are wise in their generation, who, without waiting for a danger signal, appeal periodically to some proved medicine which can be implicitly trusted to cleanse and renovate the marvellous mechanism of the human system? At no time since the days of Adam have breadwinners, whether man or woman, stood in such pressing need as they do now-a-days of a sure, convenient, and at the same time perfectly harmless antidote against brain fag, irritability, and drooping spirits. Well, to balance the bitters, you will generally, even in this hard world, find the genuine sweets somewhere, and undoubtedly it is just here where **BEECHAM'S PILLS** come cheerfully, and cheaply to the rescue. A remedy always pleasantly speedy—for we have no time to rest by the way—certain in its curative power, safe and gentle in its action, and permanent in its results, is it any wonder that BEECHAM'S PILLS have found, and are ever finding, their way into the waistcoat pocket of every wise man, and into the cupboards of every thoughtful woman, maid or matron? BEECHAM'S PILLS have long been prized for their distinct virtue of pleasingly appealing to the brain *via* the stomach, and by dispersing all "cobwebs," at once fitting us to face the struggle of modern life. Vast numbers owe their good health to BEECHAM'S PILLS, nay more, we repeat the old, bold, but honest statement that BEECHAM'S PILLS save thousands of lives yearly. Therefore, we consider the forcible assertion that first caught your eye on this page to be the plain truth, viz.—that "*in these days of high pressure,*" BEECHAM'S PILLS

ARE AN ABSOLUTE NECESSITY.

*The heading for this Beechams advert **In These Days of High Pressure** could be the 1990s – not the 1890s.*

wonderful for piles! Yes, all these remedies cured from one medication. Homocea Embrocation was described as: *Absolutely the best thing of its kind in the world* and Homocea Soap they claimed *is the finest and best soap ever made.*

How could you refuse to try **Scrubb's Cloudy Ammonia**? (*See previous page*) with such a variety of uses – *Refreshing as a Turkish Bath, Splendid Cleansing Preparation for the Hair, Removes Stains from Clothing, Restores the Colour to Carpets, Cleans Silver Plate and Jewellery, Softens Hard Water and is So Vivifying after Football, Motoring and other Sports.* [Would you try it in your bath! Today there would be at least six different products to fulfill the claims of the advertisement].

Mortimer's Rheumatic Oil was produced by JL Mortimer of Seacombe and was described as *possessed of most powerful virtuse, and produced from an article hitherto unknown to science.* One of their advertising gimics was the use of the Royal Coat of Arms to make it look as though the product was patronised by the Royal Family (*see advert on this page*). This was in fact just to confirm the product was patented.

Some products such as **Beechams Powders** (*see advertisement on this page*) have stood the test of time and are available today – over 100 years since being introduced.

The heading for their advert *In These Days of High Pressure* would have been suitable for today but was in fact taken from the 1890s – so some things don't change!

Some local chemists produced their own medicines which were reasonably priced and more likely to cure than the quack ones were.

George Wilson, Dispensing Chemist of 403 Poulton Road Poulton, advertised his 'Tonic Elixir' and 'S. & L. Pills' in a picture postcard promotion (*see page one*).

Another chemist well known locally for his own cures was Tottles Pharmacy of 224 Liscard Road, Liscard (*see photograph of shop on this page*). Mr Tottles' products included 'Tottles Bronchine' for coughs, colds, catarrh etc. and 'Tottles Pinol Creosote' which when inhaled from a handkerchief also cured coughs, colds and catarrh etc. Both items retailed at one shilling per bottle (5p). They also advertised their 'dark room' which could be used by amateur photographers.

One of the problems the customer had was to decide which of the medical advertisements were genuine and which were 'quack' when quite often the 'quack' medicines were the more plausible. However, there was the *Truth,* a weekly investigative magazine which also produced the *Truth Annual Cautionary List* of 128 pages detailing the people, companies and organisations covered by their weekly publication during the preceding two years. Ironically Dr Crippen was mentioned in the 1910 edition, the year in which he was hung for the murder of his wife.

One Hundred years on there are still plausible sounding 'quack' medicines marketed and customers willing to part with their money.

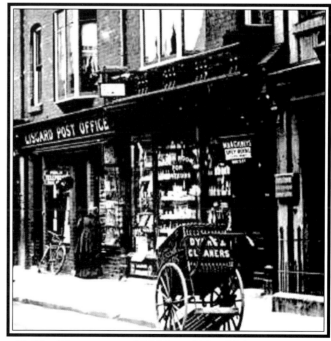

Tottles Pharmacy, at 224 Liscard Road Liscard, can be seen behind the handcart belonging to Davis & Sons, Dyers & Cleaners. Tottles were well known locally for their 'own brand' medicines (*see this page*).

Wallasey Medical Society

The Wallasey Medical Society was formed in 1910 by local doctors. There were nine founder members and the society was known as *The Society of Aphasics*. The original intention of the society was to debate topics at each other's houses. There were weekly meetings, over the winter months. The society met fourteen times over the winter of 1911 and into 1912. The minutes for 1910 do not appear to still exist but the 1911 minutes record the fact that the society had a successful 1910. It was noted that *the educational value of the society has, perhaps, not been as great as was anticipated, but as a factor in increasing and satisfying the mutual good fellowship among the members, it has been an unqualified success. That it will continue to flourish as time goes on, and that membership will be eagerly sought as opportunity arises, seems to be assured; for the regret with which the proceedings are temporarily abandoned, and the pleasure with which the meetings are resumed, are sufficient guarantee that it provides a real and sustained enjoyment.*

There were twenty rules for members to observe, including:

1X. The principals of a debate shall speak for not less than fifteen minutes and not more than thirty minutes.

X. Each member present shall speak for at least five minutes and may continue for ten minutes.

X11. A member failing to speak for the minimum time allotted must remain standing until the expiration of that time.

X1V. A fine will be inflicted upon a member if absent from three successive meetings.

XV111. Absolute secrecy shall be observed.

Members also had to agree to *submit to the ceremony of initiation laid down.* One automatically ceased to be a member on marriage! In 1912 it was unanimously agreed that there be a form of re-initiation for those members who, after matrimony, applied for re-admission to the society.

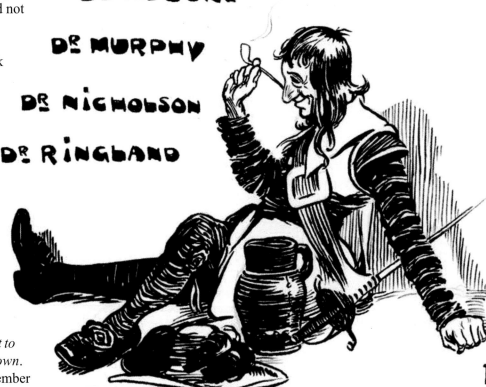

MEMBERS

DR BARRY

DR BROWN

DR DONNELL

DR LLOYD

DR LYBURN

DR McGUNE

DR MURPHY

DR NICHOLSON

DR RINGLAND

List of the Wallasey Medical Society founder members taken from the Minute Book of 1911.

By 1912 the rigours of debating led to a proposal that the society should be of a purely social character and it shall not be incumbent of any member to address the meeting. This proposal was not accepted by the majority but it was agreed that the meetings would be of a semi-social character, beginning at 8.45pm and becoming entirely social and informal after 10pm.

This was obviously a good long term decision - the Wallasey Medical Society continues to meet to this day.